RED LIGHT THERAPY

MIRACLE MEDICINE

- SECOND EDITION -

MARK SLOAN

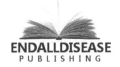

ENDALLDISEASE
PUBLISHING

RED LIGHT THERAPY: MIRACLE MEDICINE

ISBN: 978-0-9947418-6-8

"Penetrating red light is possibly the fundamental anti-stress factor for all organisms."

- Dr. Raymond Peat

CONTENTS

INTRODUCTION

WHAT IF THERE WAS A form of therapy that could correct *the root cause* of virtually all diseases and conditions known to man? What if that same therapy was also inexpensive and had literally no negative side effects? Sounds too good to be true, right? I'm here to tell you this miraculous therapy *does* exist. It's called red and near-infrared light therapy – and I wrote this book to tell you all about it.

Whether you want to reduce pain from an old injury, melt fat off your waist, hips and buttocks, get the edge over your competition by improving athletic performance, reduce anxiety and depression, boost your brain function so you can accomplish more in a day, or look and feel years younger, red light therapy is for you.

In recent years, scientific research has uncovered some fascinating information regarding the nature of disease and exactly what initiates the disease process in the first place. Soon I will describe in detail exactly how a single therapy could be so useful for such a wide variety of ailments, but for now I'll give you a brief explanation until you reach that part of the book.

The human body is a large collection of cells – trillions and trillions of them. And the most simplistic way of understanding health is to understand cellular health. Either your cells are working or they are not. When cells have everything they need to function properly, they are healthy. And if all your cells have everything they need to function properly, you as an organism, are also healthy.

The key to putting an end to most chronic degenerative diseases then is to understand exactly what cells need to function properly and why. Focusing on understanding cellular health and what it takes to keep a cell healthy is the best approach because there are a finite amount of things that one needs to learn in order to make that happen. Red light can be thought of as one of many essential nutrients required by every cell in your body.

By the time you're done reading this book you will understand exactly how the light interacts with cells and how that interaction leads to better cellular health.

WHAT IS RED LIGHT THERAPY?

Red light therapy is a form of therapy that delivers energy to cells by applying a range of visible and invisible wavelengths of light. Other names for red light therapy include low-level laser therapy (LLLT), low intensity light therapy (LILT), phototherapy, photobiostimulation, biostimulation (BIOS), photobiomodulation, photonic stimulation, among others.

Red light therapy is an FDA approved treatment for acne, muscle and joint pain, arthritis, compromised blood circulation,[1] and for reversing hair loss.[2] When you explore the 50,000+ scientific and clinical studies conducted on red light therapy to date, you'll find that no matter which disease a person has, they can probably benefit enormously from red and near-infrared light.

Red light therapy has been proven effective for a wide range of conditions including anti-aging, pain relief, cognitive enhancement, fat reduction, smoking cessation, wound healing, increasing bone density, increasing testosterone, anxiety and depression, building muscle, acne, hair loss, and many more indications that we will soon explore in complete detail.

Near-infrared light is another form of electromagnetic radiation that is similar to red light in both frequency and its beneficial biological effects.

This book is as much about near-infrared light therapy as it is red light therapy. Anytime I refer to 'red light therapy' during this writing, I am also referring to near-infrared light therapy, since they work in virtually the same way. In the following chapters, I'll outline the differences and similarities between the two.

While it was once believed that the beneficial effects of red and near-infrared light could only be obtained using expensive laser devices, it has since been established that inexpensive LEDs (light emitting diodes) can provide the same remarkable benefits at a fraction of the cost.

This means that no longer does a person have to pay large amounts of money to receive red lasers in a clinical setting. Instead, it is within reach of most people to purchase their own devices to use from the comfort of their own homes.

Near-infrared and red light therapies have virtually no adverse side effects and have a mountain of evidence supporting their remarkable therapeutic properties.

MODERN MEDICAL FAILURE

Prescription drugs are the 3rd leading cause of death after heart disease and cancer, according to Danish physician and medical researcher Peter C. Gøtzsche in 2016.[3] But prescription drugs are just one of a number of ways the medical industry ends up killing the very customers it's trying to help. Unnecessary surgeries, doctor-induced errors and X-rays are a few more.

It's time that we ask ourselves the question: Is the medical industry helping us or harming us? Remember, the only industries that survive are the ones we support.

A 2000 study by Dr. Barbara Starfield published in the *Journal of the American Medical Association* found that

"America's healthcare system is the third leading cause of death."[4] Then in 2003, for the first time ever, Dr. Gary Null and his team of researchers analyzed *all* of the existing literature on injury and death caused by mainstream medicine and came to an even more startling conclusion. "It is now evident that the American medical system is the leading cause of death and injury in the US," they wrote.[5]

It's plain to see from the evidence that our medical system is doing us far more harm than good. I think we owe it to our children and to future generations to deal with this problem instead of avoiding it and passing the burden onto them.

The beautiful thing about acknowledging this fact is that it means we are now on a journey of discovery; a learning adventure to find out if we can find better therapies and health strategies for ourselves that can replace the existing ones. Red light therapy represents a revolution in medicine and the day will come when it can be found in every household.

THE RISE OF NATURAL THERAPIES

It's time that we as a society move beyond most of the existing drug and surgical-based interventions onto new forms of therapy. Therapies that *actually* work and don't harm or kill people in the process of healing should be our goal, and it's my intention in this book to show you that red light therapy is and will forever be one of our best and brightest options.

Red light therapy has the potential to largely free humankind from expensive, damaging drugs that don't work - by transferring the power to heal from greed-driven corporations into the hands of the people, where it belongs. As people become more informed and begin investing only in medicines that deliver more benefit than harm, we will see the entire world change – quickly and painlessly – almost overnight. As with any product that sits on a shelf unpurchased, it will eventually cease being produced.

I wrote this book because I've experienced the benefits of red light therapy first-hand, and I now feel compelled to tell the world and help others do the same. The repair and enhancement of my brain function, sexual function, thyroid and overall health due to light therapy have been nothing short of miraculous.

Red light therapy isn't a cure for disease, but by optimizing cellular function, supporting the immune system and healing process, there are probably no diseases or conditions that cannot benefit from it.

It's my goal in writing this book to make the most complete resource on red light therapy ever written. One that is based on scientific evidence yet can be easily understood by anybody of any age.

It's time to bring the power to heal back into the hands of the people where it belongs, and where it will remain, until the end of time.

One thing I'd like to ask before we get started is that after you're done reading this book please remember to leave a quick review on Amazon. I read all the reviews myself and your feedback will help this book tremendously.

Thanks again for reading, and let's get started!

SECOND EDITION UPDATES

WHEN RED LIGHT THERAPY: MIRACLE Medicine was first published in May 2018, I asked readers to let me know what they would like to learn about red light therapy that wasn't covered in the book. Since then I've gotten feedback from a number of people, both in the form of emails and in book reviews on Amazon. In this second edition, I have added four new chapters, new professional artwork and bonus information all of which make this resource *even more* practical, scientific and complete. Thank you for being a part of the evolution of this book.

Interestingly, while this was the first book ever published on red light therapy for the layperson, within just a couple of months of its publication there have been swarms of kindle ebooks published on the same subject.

One author even decided to hijack the background image from the cover of this book (ebook edition) and use it on his own. The fact that virtually all of these phantom red light therapy publications have gotten almost exclusively 1-star reviews says a lot about their contents and the intention of their authors. I'd like to thank these individuals personally for making the book you hold in your hands shine even brighter, and for helping make it a 6x International #1 bestseller in the world's largest bookstore.

In this second edition, the following updates have been added:

How to use red light therapy at home: A reader named Stacy asked for more practical information on how to use red light therapy at home. In response to her request I have written a brand new chapter outlining the most practical and important advice for at-home RLT that will help you achieve the greatest possible results from red light therapy. This includes keeping sessions simple and positioning your body in a way that is comfortable and maximizes the number of cells reached by the light. I've also included a custom piece of artwork to illustrate the ideal body and light position for red light therapy.

The #1 Biggest Mistake People Make Using Red Light: A number of people have come to me frustrated with the lack of results they'd experienced using red light therapy. I asked them to describe their protocol to me and time and time again I found the same major mistake. After getting them to change just one thing about their method, they often experienced remarkable healing. In this chapter I will share with you my #1 most powerful strategy for maximizing your success with red light therapy.

Remarkable Success Stories: In recent months, my inbox has been flooded with testimonials from people who have experienced healing from red light therapy. It's one thing to observe the proven benefits of red light therapy by reading scientific studies, but when people actually begin using red light therapy and experience life-changing, 'impossible' results it becomes even more real and exciting. In this chapter I share some testimonials of people whose health and lives have been powerfully transformed through the use of red light therapy. If you ever had any doubts that red light therapy was as good as the science says it is, this will put your doubts to rest.

Bonus: 2 Proven Ways to Accelerate Healing: No matter how effective any given medicine is, it can always be improved. In this chapter I share with you two scientifically proven strategies to synergistically enhance the tissue healing capacity of red light.

Bonus Q&A: A number of questions have been added and answered including the use of red light on skin following laser hair removal, red light for rosacea and also a specific red light therapy protocol for improving vision.

Nothing can stop the revolution in the world that is now taking place with increased awareness and use of red light therapy. It's for this reason that writing this book has been such a pleasure. Nothing feels better than reducing the suffering in people's lives and in the world. The benefit that one person receives from red light therapy benefits us all. When one of us heals, we all heal.

Thanks again for reading and I hope you find the healing you've been searching for.

PART I

THE SCIENCE

CHAPTER 1

HISTORY

SINCE THE DAWN OF TIME, the medicinal properties of light have been recognized and utilized for healing. Ancient Egyptians constructed solariums fitted with colored glass to harness specific colors of the visible spectrum to heal disease.

Early use by the Greeks and Romans emphasized the thermal effects of light. Heat is beneficial for different reasons than red light, but thermal energy can be looked at as therapeutic in the same way as a sauna or a hot bath.

In 1903, Neils Ryberg Finsen was awarded the Nobel Prize in Medicine for successfully utilizing Ultraviolet light for treating tuberculosis.[1] Ultraviolet light is a type of solar radiation that interacts with cholesterol in the skin to help the body produce vitamin D. If a person is deficient in vitamin D, a large dose of it obtained by UV light can do wondrous things for a person's health. Today, Finsen is recognized as the father of modern phototherapy.

In 1910, American medical doctor John Harvey Kellogg published a book called *Light Therapeutics,* which documented his experiences healing people using incandescent light bulbs and arc lights. According to Dr. Kellogg in his book, light therapy is effective for diabetes, obesity, chronic fatigue, insomnia, baldness, cachexia and many other health problems.

In 1904, two more influential volumes on light therapy were published: *Light energy, its physics, physiological action and therapeutic applications* by Margaret A. Cleaves and *Elements of general radio-therapy for practitioners* by Leopold Freund. All three books mentioned above can be found for free online.

In the decades that followed, interest in the medicinal effects of light faded and was replaced by modern medical drug and surgical based treatments... that is, until the invention of the laser.

THE BIRTH OF THE L.A.S.E.R (LIGHT AMPLIFICATION BY STIMULATED EMISSION BY RADIATION)

The laser was invented in 1960 by American Physicist Theodore H. Maiman, but it wasn't until 1967 when Hungarian physician and surgeon Endre Mester (1903-

1984) discovered that the laser had significant therapeutic value.[2]

The ruby laser was the first laser device ever built. The image below depicts the ruby laser pumping cavity, both assembled and disassembled.

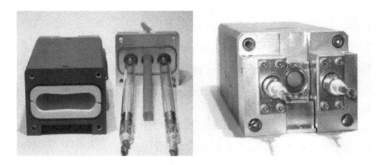

The Ruby Laser

Working at Semmelweis University in Budapest, Hungary, Dr. Mester accidentally discovered that low-level ruby laser light could regrow hair in mice. During an experiment in which he was attempting to replicate a previous study that found red laser light could shrink tumors in mice, Mester noticed that hair grew back more quickly on the treated mice than on the untreated mice.[3]

Dr. Mester went on to discover that laser light could also accelerate the healing process in mice.[4] Following this discovery, he founded the *Laser Research Center* at the Semmelweiss Medical University in Budapest in 1974, where he worked for the remainder of his life.

Adam Mester, Dr. Andre Mester's son, was reported in an article by *New Scientist* in 1987 - some 20 years after his father's discovery - to have been using lasers on 'otherwise incurable' ulcers. "He takes patients referred by other specialists who can do no more for them," the article reads. "Of the 1300 treated so far, he has achieved complete healing in 80 percent and partial healing in 15 percent."[5]

Interestingly, due to a lack of understanding of how lasers imparted their beneficial effects, many scientists and physicians at the time had attributed it to "magic".

In North America, red light research didn't begin to take hold until around the year 2000. Since then, publishing activity has grown almost exponentially, particularly in the most recent years.

A quick search on PubMed of the various terms describing light therapy renders over 50,000 published scientific and clinical studies:

- Phototherapy = 37,785 studies

- Photobiomodulation = 510 studies

- Photostimulation = 1,067 studies

- Lllt = 5,139 studies

- Low-level laser therapy = 5,910 studies

- Near-infrared light = 8,431 studies

Now that we understand more about the history of light therapy, let's look at what exactly red and near-infrared light are.

CHAPTER 2

RED & NEAR-INFRARED RADIATION

MOST PEOPLE ARE AWARE THAT sunlight is a rich source of UVB radiation, which stimulates the production of vitamin D and protects us from numerous ailments such as autoimmune disorders, various types of cancer and cardiovascular disease.[1]

What most people aren't aware of is the other significant source of therapeutic radiation the sun offers us: Light emitted in the red and near-infrared ends of the spectrum. Dr. Ray Peat has theorized that red and near-infrared light could be "the fundamental anti-stress factor for all organisms." This means that, far more than just a beneficial nutrient for humans, red light is a factor that's essential for the health of literally every living creature on earth, including plants.

While an excess of ultraviolet light can cause sunburn, red and near-infrared light protect the skin from sunburn.

A FEW WORDS ON TANNING BEDS

Understanding more about the radiation emitted from tanning beds can help put solar radiation and red light therapy into context.

Typical tanning beds give off 95% light in the UVA spectrum and only 5% UVB, which is of the type that converts cholesterol in the skin into Vitamin D.

Unlike the sun, tanning beds emit only the damaging frequencies with no protective red or near-infrared light. Without red and near-infrared light to help protect against ultraviolet exposure, ultraviolet light becomes increasingly more damaging.

Ultraviolet light causes damage in the same way as ionizing radiation from X-rays or radiotherapy. The only difference is that when you get a sunburn you're only being burnt on the surface of your skin, whereas a cancer patient who receives radiotherapy will be burnt through their entire body.

The fact that tanning beds emit ionizing ultraviolet radiation without red or near-infrared light is why they are considered dangerous and known to cause cancer.

I think it's useful to mention that tanning beds can be made safer and more medicinal by replacing around 60%

of their UV bulbs with bulbs in the red or near-infrared end of the spectrum. This will, in effect, offer a more balanced assortment of radiation that more closely approximates natural sunlight.

WHAT IS RED LIGHT?

Shine light through a prism and the light will fragment into all the colors that makeup the visible spectrum of light, including green, blue, purple, yellow, orange and red. Most of us have done this experiment, but for those of us who haven't here is an illustration of how it will look.

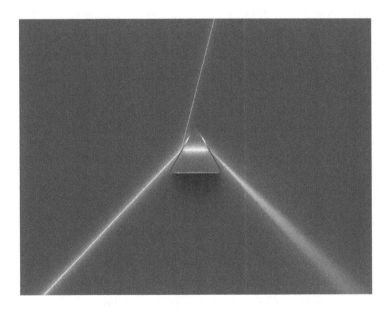

Red light is a form of radiation that's visible to the human eye and exists between 600-700 nanometers in wavelength.

Most wavelengths of light, such as ultraviolet, blue or green light, don't penetrate the skin deeply at all and are instead absorbed by the surface layers of skin. Some colors of light, like blue, have the opposite effect of red light on cellular health. Unlike other colors, red light easily penetrates skin, which makes it useful therapeutically for reaching cells and tissues deep inside the body.

THE CELL PHONE FLASHLIGHT EXPERIMENT

To witness the unique ability of red light to penetrate deeply into body tissues, here is an interesting experiment you can try which I learned from Finnish health researcher Vladimir Heiskanen in his comprehensive paper on red and near-infrared light therapy.[2]

Instructions:

Take out your mobile phone and load the flashlight application.

Next, hold the tip of your finger directly against the light and look at your finger. What do you see?

Although your mobile phone flashlight emits blue, green and red light - only the red light penetrates all the way through your finger. Look at the red glow!

Red light ranges in wavelength from about 620-700 nanometers (nm).

The following is a diagram of both visible and invisible wavelengths electromagnetic radiation and the colors they create when perceived by the human eye.

Visible Spectrum of Light

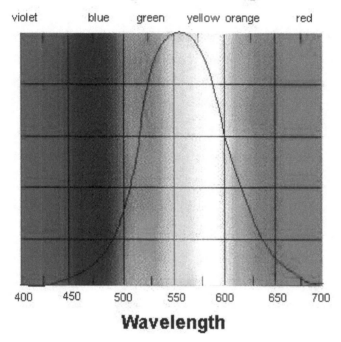

WHAT IS NEAR-INFRARED LIGHT?

Every time we feel heat from the sun on our skin or the warmth of a campfire we are experiencing infrared light.

The human eye is limited to seeing wavelengths of light ranging between 400-700 nanometers, and anything below or above that, such as infrared light, remains invisible or light-pink. Interestingly, although invisible to the human eye, the human body can feel parts of the electromagnetic spectrum that cannot be seen, such as infrared.

The infrared spectrum ranges from 700 nm – 1 mm (10,000nm) and is actually divided up into near-infrared, middle-infrared, and far-infrared.

There are many conflicting opinions as to where near, middle and far-infrareds begin and end. The following wavelengths are from a paper written by Hong Kong scientist Cheah Kok Wai called *The Fundamentals of Far-Infrared*:[3]

- **Near-Infrared** (also called Infrared-A or IR-A) = 700nm - 1400nm

- **Mid-Infrared** (also called Infrared-B or IR-B) = 1,400nm - 3,000nm

- **Far-Infrared** (also called Infrared-C or IR-C) = 3,000nm - 1mm

The most therapeutic wavelengths of infrared light range from 700nm to about 1400nm.

RED VS. NEAR-INFRARED LIGHT

The physiological effects of red and near-infrared light in the body occur in similar ways. For therapeutic applications, the primary difference between the two is that near-infrared light penetrates more deeply into the body than red light, meaning it can reach and benefit cells that red light cannot. That being said, every session with red light benefits the entire body, because factors released from cells which receive red light promote proper function in cells adjacent to them. Furthermore, blood cells also absorb red light, so as it passes the area of the body being exposed to red light, the light absorbed will then travel through the bloodstream and end up nourishing cells in other regions of the body. This means that all red light sessions reward the entire body as a whole, or *holistically*.

While red light is often used for superficial applications like skin health, for example acne, near-infrared light can be used for both the skin and to reach tissues residing deeper within the body.

The wavelengths of red and near-infrared light shown to be the most therapeutic in scientific research are as follows:

MAXIMAL THERAPEUTIC RANGE	
Red Light	620-700nm
Near-Infrared	700-1000nm

Even within these effective ranges of red and near-infrared light, some wavelengths have been found to be more or less beneficial than others. The four most efficiently absorbed wavelengths of red and near-infrared light have been found to be 620nm, 670nm, 760nm and 830nm.

Many light therapy devices today emit multiple wavelengths of either red or infrared light and some even combine both red and infrared wavelengths into a single device.

For certain skin conditions, some evidence suggests red light might be more beneficial than near-infrared light. For all practical purposes, near-infrared light or a combination of red and near-infrared light is probably ideal.

I use a light therapy device that contains both red and near-infrared LEDs so I receive the best of both worlds; a 50/50 application of visible red and invisible near-infrared light. I love watching the room light up with red light during sessions, which is one of the reasons I prefer a combination device over solely near-infrared light.

RED RADIATION REJUVENATION

Both red and near-infrared radiation are essential for all biological life and can be obtained by exposing the body to sunlight. Although UVB radiation, which can also be obtained through sunlight, is essential for humans to produce Vitamin D, too much can cause burning of the skin.

Red and near-infrared radiation protect the body from damaging radiation and bolster energy production inside every cell with which they interact.

Summary:

Red and near-infrared light are similar in wavelength, impart their benefits similarly, and the primary difference between the two is that near-infrared radiation penetrates deeper into body tissues than red light.

CHAPTER 3

THE SCIENCE OF LIGHT THERAPY

RUSSIAN SCIENTISTS WERE THE FIRST to explore and document the health effects of red light scientifically in the early 1900s. Some of the most commonly known benefits of red light today in the United States had already been discovered almost 100 years ago by Russian researchers.

It wasn't until around the year 2000 that we saw an explosion of interest in red light research in western countries like the United States. And since then, the amount of publishing activity on the subject has increased almost exponentially. To date there have been over

50,000 published papers on red and near-infrared light therapies.

Over the past 100 years, infrared and red light therapies have been studied extensively on human beings and many other animals for dozens of diseases and conditions. Animals and creatures like rats,[1] mice,[2] rabbits,[3] mini-pigs,[4] dogs,[5] monkeys,[6] pigs,[7] sheep,[8] horses,[9] cows,[10] cats,[11] sand rats,[12] gerbils,[13] guinea pigs,[14] frogs,[15] bumblebees,[16] fruit flies,[17] sea urchin larvae,[18] snails,[19] roundworms,[20] earthworms[21] and flat worms[22] have all shown to benefit from red light. When given the option, many of these animals prefer being in the field of red light; instead of avoiding it or acting indifferent, they home to it in delight like bears to a honey bee hive.

As it turns out, the cellular metabolic processes for humans and other creatures are very similar, which is why we see consistently similar health benefits among different species.

DISEASES AND CONDITIONS AFFECTED BY RED LIGHT

The following is a list of diseases and conditions which scientific evidence shows can benefit from red and near-infrared light. Some of these studies have been well-established through scientific reviews and meta-analysis and others are said to be controversial and more research may be necessary.

However, keep in mind that just because something may be controversial doesn't mean it's not true. I think it's very likely that red light can benefit every single condition below, and many more that aren't in the list because they haven't yet been studied.

- Achilles Tendinitis[23-24]
- Achilles Tendinopathy[25-26]
- Acne[27-29]
- Addiction[30]
- Amblyopia[31]
- Age-Related Macular Degeneration[32-33]
- Alzheimer's Disease[34]
- Aphthous Ulcers[35-37]
- Bell's Palsy[38-40]
- Bone Fractures[41-43]
- Burn Scars[44]
- Burning Mouth Syndrome[45-46]
- Carpal Tunnel Syndrome[47-48]
- Cellulite[49]
- Chronic Joint Disorders[50]
- Cognitive Enhancement[51-54]
- Cold Sores (herpes labialis)[55-56]
- COPD[57]
- Dental Implant Stability[58]
- Dentin Hypersensitivity[59]
- Depression[60-62]
- Diabetic Foot Ulcer[63-64]

- Dry Mouth (xerostomy)[65-67]
- Dysmenorrhea[68-69]
- Elbow Tendinopathy (Tennis Elbow)[70]
- Exercise Performance and Recovery[71-75]
- Fibromyalgia[76-77]
- Frozen Shoulder[78]
- Glaucoma[79]
- Hair Loss (alopecia)[80-81]
- Hand-foot-and-mouth disease[82]
- Hypothyroidism[83-85]
- Lichen Planus[86]
- Low Back Pain[87-89]
- Lymphedema[90-92]
- Maxillary Sinusitis[93]
- Meniscal Pathology[94]
- Muscle Growth[95-96]
- Muscle Pain[97]
- Neck Pain[98-99]
- Neuropathic Foot Ulcer[100]
- Nipple Pain (from Breastfeeding)[101-102]
- Obesity[103-105]
- Oral Mucositis[106-108]
- Orthodontic Pain[109-111]
- Orthodontic Tooth Movement[112]
- Osteoarthritis[113-115]
- Osteoporosis (Bone Loss)[116-117]

- Pain[118-119]
- Periodontitis (Gum Disease)[120]
- Postherpetic Neuralgia[121]
- Pressure Ulcer[122-123]
- Radation Dermatitis[124-126]
- Raynaud's Phenomenon[127]
- Restenosis[128]
- Rheumatoid Arthritis[129-131]
- Shoulder Tendinopathy[132]
- Skin Aging[133-134]
- Sternotomy Incision Repair[135-137]
- Stroke[138-140]
- Sunburn Prevention[141]
- Temporomandibular Disorders[142]
- Tendinopathy[143]
- Testosterone Deficiency[144]
- Toenail Fungus[145-147]
- Traumatic Brain Injury[148-149]
- Venous Leg Ulcers[150]
- Vitiligo[151-152]
- Wound Healing[153-155]

Despite the immense number of scientific papers published on red and near-infrared light, there is still much to be learned and research at universities and other institutions continues to this day.

To be clear though, no more research is needed for us to gain the remarkable benefits of red light. We know red light is safe and effective - and now it's time to put it to use.

RED LIGHT FOR HEALING & REGENERATION

The overall health of your body is dependent on its supply of energy. That's because every single critical process that takes place inside your body – from repair and regeneration to detoxification to immunity to the blinking of your eyes and the beating of your heart – all require energy to be successfully orchestrated.

If you woke up one day and literally had no energy available, you wouldn't rise up out of bed and eventually you would die. The same thing can be said for the cells that make up the body; they also require energy for their survival. And in fact, your body gets its energy from your individual cells - so if your cells are energized and healthy, your body is energized and healthy.

Within cells are tiny energy-producing 'power plants' called mitochondria, which are the source of the energy for your cells and for your body as a whole.

When mitochondria inside a cell have everything they need to produce energy efficiently, that cell is healthy. And when the majority of your cells have everything the mitochondria within them need to produce energy efficiently, your body is healthy.

The substances needed for efficient energy production can be called nutrients, almost all of which can be obtained through dietary means. One of the few nutrients which are essential for efficient energy production that cannot be obtained through dietary means is red light.

Soon we will explore in greater detail the physiological effects of red light, but before we do, let's take a look at 10 of the most remarkable benefits of red light therapy.

CHAPTER 4

TOP 10 PROVEN BENEFITS OF RED LIGHT

NOW THAT YOU'VE SEEN THE long list of diseases and conditions that red and near-infrared light therapy can benefit, let's go a little more in depth into some of them. The findings of some of these studies are remarkable, and they will give you a good indication of how powerful of a remedy red light is and what it can do for you.

Here is my top 10 list of some of the most common ailments for which red and near-infrared light therapies show enormous potential.

BENEFIT #10:
MELT YOUR BELLY FAT

According to the Centre for Disease Control (the CDC), more than one-third (36.5%) of U.S. adults are obese. Obese people have an increased risk of a number of conditions including heart disease, stroke, type 2 diabetes and cancer, so correcting this condition is vital for long term health.[1]

Another benefit of fat reduction in an obese person is the money saved on medical costs every year. How much money? The medical costs for people who have obesity are $1,429 higher per year than those of 'normal' weight.[1]

So there you have it – reducing obesity can not only improve the health of the individual, but it can reduce their cost of living as well as the stress associated with having to spend more money on medical bills.

There are no shortages of people, programs and devices claiming they can help people burn fat – but we all know many of them turn out to be fraudulent and don't actually work. Others can help you lose weight but they do so in ways that are excessively stressful and unhealthy.

Can red and near-infrared light therapies help you safely burn fat? The following evidence suggests it can, and more efficiently than most people would imagine.

In 2015, a team of researchers from the Federal University of São Paulo, Brazil tested the effects of near-infrared light (808nm) on 64 obese women randomly assigned to one of two groups: Exercise (aerobic &

resistance) training + phototherapy or exercise (aerobic & resistance) training + no phototherapy. The study took place over a 20 week period, during which both groups of obese women underwent exercise training 3-times a week. At the end of each training session, one group of women received light therapy and the other did not.

The results?

Remarkably, the women who received the near-infrared light therapy following exercise *doubled* the amount of fat loss compared to exercise alone. Additionally, the women in the exercise + phototherapy group were reported to have a greater increase in skeletal muscle mass than the placebo group.[2]

Other studies have reported similar findings in obese people who combined exercise with red light therapy,[3-4] but even studies that *did not* include exercise have reported significant fat reduction from red light therapy alone.[5-6]

Scientists from George Washington University conducted an independent physician-led trial in 2013 to test the ability of red laser light (635nm) to reduce fat on the waist, hips and thighs of obese individuals. Red light was administered to 8 obese patients and consisted of 20 minute sessions every second day for two weeks. When researchers assessed the patients three weeks after the trial began (one week after sessions ended) the results were remarkable. "Compared with baseline, a statistically significant 2.99in. (7.59cm) mean loss was observed at the post-procedure evaluation point."

Translation: Patients lost 3 inches of fat in just two weeks of red light therapy.[6]

BENEFIT #9:
WOUND REPAIR

Whether it's from an accident during physical activity or chemical pollutants in our food and environment, we all sustain injuries regularly. Anything that can fortify the body's innate healing process will allow it to focus its available energy on the maintenance of health.

Dr. Harry Whelan from the Medical College of Wisconsin has been studying red light in cell cultures and on humans for decades. His work in the laboratory has shown that skin and muscle cells grown in cultures and exposed to LED infrared light grow 150-200% faster than control cultures not stimulated by the light.[7]

Working with Naval doctors in Norfolk, Virginia and San Diego California to nurse injured soldiers, Dr. Whelan and his team found that soldiers with musculoskeletal training injuries who were administered red light improved by 40%.[7]

In 2000, Dr. Whelan concluded after many years of research that "The near-infrared light emitted by these LEDs seems to be perfect for increasing energy inside cells. This means whether you're on Earth in a hospital, working in a submarine under the sea or on your way to Mars inside a spaceship, the LEDs boost energy to the cells and accelerate healing."

A review of the scientific literature reveals there are literally dozens of other studies evidencing the powerful wound-healing benefits of red light.[8]

In 2014, a group of scientists from three universities in Brazil conducted a scientific review of the effects of red light on wound healing. After reviewing a total of 68 studies, most of which were conducted on animals using wavelengths ranging from 632 to 830 nm, the study concluded "...phototherapy, either by LASER or LED, is an effective therapeutic modality to promote healing of skin wounds."[9]

No matter how you have been wounded, red light therapy has the capacity to improve the body's healing process.

BENEFIT #8:
INCREASED BONE DENSITY

Bone density and the ability of the body to build new bone is important for people recovering from injuries. It's also important for elderly people since our bones tend to progressively become weaker with age. Anybody who isn't sick and wants to remain physically active for as much of their lives as possible has an interest in building and maintaining strong, healthy bones.

The restorative effects of red and near-infrared light on bone have been demonstrated in many laboratory studies.

In 2013, researchers from São Paulo, Brazil studied the effects of red and near-infrared light on the healing of rat bones. First, a piece of bone was sliced off the upper leg (osteotomy) of 45 rats, which were then split into three groups: Group 1 received no light, group 2 was administered red light (660-690nm) and group 3 was exposed to near-infrared light (790-830nm).

The study found "a significant increase in the degree of mineralization (gray level) in both groups treated with the laser after 7 days" and interestingly, "after 14 days, only the group treated with laser therapy in the infrared spectrum showed higher bone density."[10]

Here are a few more studies on light therapy for bone health and their conclusions.

2003 study conclusion:

"We conclude that LLLT had a positive effect on the repair of bone defects implanted with inorganic bovine bone."[11]

2006 study conclusion:

"The results of our studies and others indicate that bone irradiated mostly with infrared (IR) wavelengths shows increased osteoblastic proliferation, collagen deposition, and bone neoformation when compared to nonirradiated bone."[12]

2008 study conclusion:

"The use of laser technology has been used to improve the clinical results of bone surgeries and to promote a more comfortable postoperative period and quicker healing."[13]

Red and near-infrared light can be used to build more robust bones in people young and old. After breaking a bone or incurring any kind of bodily injury, near-infrared and red light therapies should be used as a first line of defense for rapid recovery.

BENEFIT #7:
INCREASE TESTOSTERONE

Throughout history, the essence of a man has been linked to his primary male hormone testosterone. At around the age of 30, testosterone levels begin to decline and this can result in a number of negative changes to a man's physical and mental health and wellbeing: Reduced sexual function, low energy levels, reduced muscle mass and increased fat, among others.[14]

When you factor in the endless environmental contaminants, stress and poor nutrition that are so common today, it's no surprise that we are seeing an epidemic of low testosterone in men the world over.[15]

In 2013, a group of Korean researchers studied the impact of testicular exposure to red (670nm) and near-infrared (808nm) laser light. The 30 male rats were split up into three groups: a control group and two groups that were exposed to either the red or near-infrared light. At the end of the 5-day trial, while untreated rats had no increase in testosterone, rats exposed to one 30-minute session of light therapy per day had significantly elevated testosterone levels. "…Serum T level was significantly increased in the 808nm wavelength group. In the 670 nm wavelength group, serum T level was also significantly increased at the same intensity of 360 J/cm2/day," concluded researchers.[16]

It's important to note that testicle tissue is one of the few tissues in the body whose function is hindered by elevated temperature. Wearing 'tighty whitey' underwear, which holds the testicles against the body, raising their temperature, is known to reduce testosterone and sperm count. The testicles need to 'dangle' and hang down, making loose-fitting boxers a better choice of underwear for men.

For this same reason, it's important to keep the light about a foot away when applying red light to the testicles. Don't let this discourage you from experimenting. The study results have been remarkable, and at the very worst, if you position your red light too close and you apply too much heating to the area, your sex drive and testosterone levels may be impeded for a short period of time before returning to baseline.

BENEFIT #6:
ENHANCE BRAIN FUNCTION

Nootropics (pronounced: no-oh-troh-picks), also called smart drugs or cognitive enhancers, have undergone a dramatic spike in popularity in recent years and are being used by many people to enhance brain functions such as memory, creativity and motivation.

The positive effects of red light on brain function are significant and well established scientifically. In fact, light in the red and near-infrared spectrums could very well be the most powerful nootropics ever discovered. Let's look at some evidence for this.

Researchers from the University of Texas applied near-infrared laser light to the foreheads of healthy volunteers and measured its effects on cognitive parameters, including attention, memory and mood in 2013. The light therapy group experienced improvements in reaction time, memory and an increase in positive emotional states at the two-week follow-up. "These data imply that transcranial laser stimulation could be used as a non-invasive and efficacious approach to increase brain functions such as those related to cognitive and emotional dimensions," wrote scientists.[17]

Another study investigated the effects of near-infrared laser light on the brain both individually and in combination with aerobic exercise. Compared to the control group, which didn't receive the light or the exercise, the American researchers concluded that phototherapy had brain-boosting effects similar to the exercise.[18]

If you're currently enrolled in school, red light can help you memorize and recall information, increase your ability to work for long periods of time and have your brain functioning optimally for tests.

Parents who administer red light on the foreheads of their young children will not only help their kids learn better, but it will allow them to more easily connect with other students and develop long lasting relationships. I'm excited to see the geniuses that arise in this world as a direct result of being raised by parents who applied red light to their brains and bodies regularly.

BENEFIT #5:
ELIMINATE ANXIETY AND DEPRESSION

Depression affects 121 million people worldwide,[19] and that's only the number of people *officially* diagnosed with it. The truth is we all experience depression at some point in our lives. And when we do, many of us turn to drugs or other drug-like behaviors that help raise dopamine levels, such as pornography, social media or video games. I know that many people long to feel the liberation associated with not having to depend on these props to cope with life.

A 2017 study on the mental health status of Americans found that more people than ever are suffering from serious mental health disorders.[20] That's 8.3 million American adults suffering from serious psychological distress, including feelings of sadness, worthlessness and restlessness.

University students – the ones who are supposed to be our smartest and healthiest leaders-of-tomorrow – experience significantly higher rates of depression than your average population, according to a 2012 scientific review.[21]

Even more troubling: "Depression is associated with high suicidality," wrote scientist M.S. Reddy in 2010. "About 50% of individuals who have committed suicide carried a primary diagnosis of depression," continued Reddy.[19]

Anxiety is even more common than depression – it's the most common mental illness in the U.S. – affecting 40 million adults age 18 and older (18.1%).[22]

Existing medical interventions for anxiety and depression are toxic, tend to numb people out and have even been implicated in causing aggressive and suicidal behavior. This, in my estimation, is due largely to a misunderstanding of the role of serotonin in the human body. However, that is a subject for another time as it's beyond the scope of this book. Clearly new and effective therapies are desperately needed to curb anxiety, depression and today's alarming rate of suicide.

Just imagine how much better life would be for us all if people had a way of melting away their feelings of anxiety and depression.

Is red light effective for anxiety and depression?

In 2009, a group of scientists from Harvard University tested the effects of near-infrared light on 10 subjects with major depression. Researchers applied the light directly to the forehead of patients in one 16 minute session. After just one session with near-infrared light, "Patients experienced highly significant reductions in both HAM-D [depression] and HAM-A [anxiety] scores following treatment, with the greatest reductions occurring at 2 weeks."[23]

Translation: Near-infrared light therapy resulted in long-lasting reductions in depression and anxiety from *just one* session.

BENEFIT #4:
ELIMINATE ACNE VULGARIS

Acne is the most widespread skin condition in the U.S., affecting up to 50 million Americans annually.[24]

People react differently to the presence of acne on their face and body, but it often results in poor self-image, depression anxiety and many times permanent physical scarring of the skin.[25]

A 2001 experiment from Queens Medical Center in Nottingham, UK found that acne was prevalent in 50% of adolescents and had "considerable impact on emotional health in this age group."[26]

Towards the end of grade school I began developing pretty severe acne. I remember how much it affected me psychologically. In reality, it wasn't nearly as bad physically as I perceived it to be, but I can remember seeing a cute girl in class or in the halls and all that was on my mind was that I needed to make sure she didn't see it. It definitely had a negative effect on my personal relationships and social interaction, and I wish I had had something better than the ineffective cream the dermatologist gave me.

At one point, the dermatologist put me on a drug called Accutane, which didn't work and made me suicidal after I stopped taking it. The drug was high-dose synthetic vitamin A, which has nothing to do with real vitamin A and is incredibly toxic. Obviously I didn't end up killing myself, but I did some things that caused me permanent damage like punching a wall, which broke a few of my knuckles. It also directly caused literally dozens of freckles to pop up over my entire body. Unfortunately those freckles were permanent and they still have a negative effect on my self-image to this day.

Anyways, a few years ago I saw an advertisement by a lawyer on television requesting that all people who had been injured by Accutane to 'call now.' I wasn't surprised to hear many other people had damaged by that horrendous drug. I didn't end up calling but I hope many people got some compensation for their negative experiences with Accutane.

Is light therapy effective for acne?

Iranian scientists compared the effects of red (630nm) and near-infrared (890nm) laser therapy on 28 patients with facial acne in 2012. Participants in the study were given light therapy on their face 2-times per week for 6 weeks and their skin conditions were then assessed. Ten weeks following light therapy, acne lesions were found to be significantly decreased in those administered red light, but the decrease wasn't significant with the near-infrared light.[27]

Thanks to the scientific discovery of red light as a remedy for acne, present and future generations of children no longer have to deal with swollen, red, painful pus-oozing pimples and all the negative implications on their psychology and social lives.

It is your duty and mine to make kids aware of red light therapy as a safe and effective remedy for acne so they know where to reach if and when pimples begin to form.

BENEFIT #3:
RELIEVE PAIN

America is a nation in pain, according to a 2015 study by researchers at the National Institutes of Health. How much pain?

Nearly 50 million American adults (11.2%) reported experiencing pain daily for the previous-three months.[28]

Some of the most common pain medications that people reach for when they are feeling pain are Tylenol, Ibuprofen or other drugs classified as Non-Steroidal Anti-Inflammatory Drugs (NSAIDS). Interestingly, all of these common painkillers have been shown to cause heart attacks, strokes and cancer, except aspirin, which actually reduces the risk of these same complications. In 2015, the FDA issued a strong warning that all NSAIDs except aspirin can trigger heart attacks and strokes.[29]

In other words, people experiencing pain are using medications which are slowly killing them. Interestingly, aspirin and red light kill pain in similar ways, by reducing an enzyme called COX-2. But more about that later. What we know for certain is that safer and more effective therapies are needed to reduce the chronic pain people are experiencing.

The following are the conclusions of a few recent publications on pain reduction using therapeutic red and near-infrared light.

2006 systematic review:

"There is strong evidence that LLLT [low-level laser therapy] modulates the inflammatory process and relieves acute pain in the short-term."[30]

2009 systematic review published in *The Lancet*:

"We show that LLLT reduces pain immediately after treatment in acute neck pain and up to 22 weeks after completion of treatment in patients with chronic neck pain."[31]

2014 review:

"[red and near-infrared] Laser causes pain relief without any side effects."[32]

It's clear from the evidence that red light therapy is an all-star in the new world of metabolic-enhancing supplements that can help reduce the pain and suffering in people's lives.

BENEFIT #2:
HAIR REGROWTH

Hair loss (alopecia) is a very common disorder, affecting more than 50% of the worldwide population.[33]

In the United States, an estimated 35 million men and 21 million women suffer from some form of hair loss, and around 40% of men will have noticeable hair loss by the age 35.[34]

If you think of each hair follicle as a hair-producing factory, then it can be said that in somebody experiencing hair loss, the factory has been shut down. In theory, the damaged hair follicles could once again produce hair. Restoring function to hair follicles is as much about tending to the needs of the follicles themselves as it is to the health of the remainder of the body.

It's important to note that hair production is not an essential function for human survival, so under stress it's one of the first things to go. Reproduction is another. If you're suffering from hair loss, it is the direct result of excess stress in your life.

When most people think about relieving stress they think meditation, yoga and breathing exercises. Stress can be psychological and these things can definitely be useful, but many potent physiological stressors are often overlooked, like exposure to chemicals, radio frequency radiation or lack of essential nutrients. Reducing stress in a multitude of ways is an effective strategy for reversing hair loss.

To date there are only two FDA-approved synthetic drugs for hair loss available from your doctor: Propecia and Rogaine. Both of these drugs have a less than 50% success rate, and potential side effects of both drugs are severe.[35]

Hair transplants are another option, but they come with a long list of unwanted side effects including itching, pain, bleeding, swelling, infections, etc. And like the available drug treatments for hair loss, the efficacy of hair transplants is feeble at best.

"I only have to venture to a major street in San Francisco to find that if there were an 'effective' treatment for baldness, a majority of men are either not aware of it, or are choosing to be bald," wrote hair-loss researcher Danny Roddy.[36]

Can red light help regrow hair?

American and Hungarian researchers conducted a review in 2014 of studies involving red and near-infrared laser therapy for hair loss. The review reports that red and near-infrared laser therapies have been demonstrated to stimulate hair growth in both mice and in men and women in a number of controlled clinical trials. "LLLT for hair growth in both men and women appears to be both safe and effective," they concluded.[33]

BENEFIT #1:
ARTHRITIS

Arthritis is a crippling ailment from which many people worldwide suffer. An estimated 22.7% of US adults were diagnosed with some form of arthritis between the years 2013-2015. That's almost 55 million people who could benefit from an effective treatment for the condition.[37]

I've never experienced arthritis myself, but one of my previous girlfriend's friends suffered from arthritis severely, and remarkably she was only 28 years old at the time. Whereas arthritis used to exist almost exclusively in elderly people, today it seems to be more prevalent among young people.

The closest thing I've experienced to arthritis was after I stubbed my finger on a basketball. I remember not being able to bend my finger for about a week due to the swelling and pain. I can hardly imagine having to deal with that immobility, pain and discomfort on a regular basis. I feel for anybody who suffers from arthritis, and I added this section to the book with you in mind.

Currently, there are dozens of different FDA-approved drugs for arthritis, all of which come with limited successes as well as their own set of potentially serious side effects.

Is red light effective for arthritis?

Dr. Michael R. Hamblin, Harvard professor from the Department of Dermatology, published a study in 2013 titled *Can Osteoarthritis Be Treated with Light?* The study experimented with the application of near-infrared laser light (810nm) on arthritis in rats. Remarkably, after inducing arthritis in the rats and administering light therapy just *one time*, inflammation was found to be significantly reduced in just 24 hours. "A single application of LLLT produced significant reductions in inflammatory cell infiltration and inflammatory cytokines 24 hours later."[38]

For people frustrated by the struggle to find a safe and effective remedy for arthritis, red light could be the answer.

What book on red light therapy would be complete without addressing the one disease that threatens human existence more than any other?

CHAPTER 5

LIGHT THERAPY FOR CANCER

ONE THING THAT MOST OF us have in common, regardless of geographic location, race, religion or gender, is that we've all been affected on a personal level by cancer. Anybody who hasn't lost a friend or family member to cancer at this point can consider themselves lucky. For me it was my mom, who died of cancer when I was 12 years old.

Like any child who has endured such a loss, the effect it had on my life was devastating. I spent years feeling broken, confused and angry about it. It wasn't until about 20 years after she died that I realized this tragedy I went through was actually my greatest opportunity. My mother gave me a story that could inspire others and an endless source of motivation that I could use to find the answers that people were literally dying to know.

It's been almost 50 years since the war on cancer has been declared and yet more people are diagnosed and dying of the disease than ever before. If you give somebody 50 years and around $500 Billion dollars in research money to find a cure for cancer and they literally come up with nothing, what do you do? You fire them and find a new approach.

About three years ago I realized that the time to sit around waiting for answers was over. It was at that very moment when I committed to researching and publishing a book about cancer. My mission was to learn everything I could and present my findings in such a way that anybody of any age could understand and apply that knowledge to their lives. I had no idea what I was going to find, but ultimately I realized that all the scientific research needed to resolve the disease of cancer had already been completed.

In 2018, after three of the most challenging years of my life, I published two books on cancer, one called *The Cancer Industry* and another called *Cancer: The Metabolic Disease Unraveled*. Both books include a combined total of over 2500 scientific and clinical references and together are undoubtedly the most thorough investigation into cancer ever written. I highly recommend you to read them. The reality is nobody needs to die of cancer anymore; all the research needed to leave the disease behind us forever has already been completed.

An industry that makes $126 Billion dollars a year will never give us answers, if those answers would mean putting itself out of business. It's up to us as individuals to understand what cancer is, and the most efficient ways to remedy it, that will forever make cancer history.

In this chapter, my goal will be to accurately and scientifically summarize the cancer problem and then show how red and near-infrared light therapy could potentially be helpful.

THE CANCER EPIDEMIC

Governments of the world tell us that 50% of people alive will develop cancer at some point in their lives. The most frightening thing about that figure is that if we are diagnosed with cancer, doctors will recommend we undergo 'treatments' which can double as weapons of war. Knives (surgery), poison (chemotherapy) and the same ionizing radiation that is emitted from nuclear bombs (radiotherapy) are all effective ways of killing enemy soldiers on the battlefield. Is it any wonder that the word cancer is probably the most feared word in the English language?

We've all seen at least somebody in our lives undergo surgery, chemotherapy and radiotherapy and then come out far worse than before. I saw it happen to my mother when I was 12 years old. As soon as she received chemotherapy, it was like she got hit by a truck. Instead of recovering, she died a few months later, and every moment from chemotherapy to death was spent in agony.

It's common sense that cutting a sick person with a knife, injecting poison into their bodies, and burning them with ionizing radiation will make their health worse. Our own human experience has validated this on endless occasions and even the scientific evidence agrees. It's time to learn from history and take action instead of ignoring it:

Dr. Hardin B Jones, professor of medical physics at the University of California, Berkeley and leading US cancer statistician for over 30 years, declared the following at a conference for the national cancer institute way back in 1969:

"My studies have proved conclusively that untreated cancer victims live up to four times longer than treated individuals. If one has cancer and opts to do nothing at all, he will live longer and feel better than if he undergoes radiation, chemotherapy or surgery, other than when used in immediate life-threatening situations."

CANCER: THE METABOLIC DISEASE

The biggest myth being taught by the cancer industry is that a cancer cell is some kind of microscopic terrorist that's intent on killing people. This concept is about as real as The Loch Ness Monster or the legendary Chupacabra. No scientific evidence has ever suggested that cancer cells or tumors have any intention of killing anyone. The idea that cancer is a genetically-mutated monster which will kill us if we don't kill it is the popular mythology perpetuated by the cancer industry. It's the only way to justify the use of knives, poisons and radiation on cancer patients.

The National Cancer Institute's own billion-dollar initiative, which was launched in 2005 and was titled *The Cancer Genome Atlas Project,* proved conclusively that not a single gene mutation - or any combination of mutations - was found to be absolutely responsible for initiating the disease.[1-5]

This is because cancer is not a genetic disease.

It's been almost 100 years since Nobel Prize-Winning scientist Dr. Otto Warburg discovered that a cancer cell was a cell with damaged mitochondria – a tiny organelle within cells that is responsible for energy production.[6] What Warburg's work has revealed to us is that a cancer cell is simply a metabolically defective/injured cell that's in need of repair.

The remarkable truth is that the cancer industry treats injuries with treatments that cause injury. That's the sum of their medical intelligence.

After *The Cancer Genome Atlas Project* proved that cancer is not a genetic disease but a metabolic one, James Watson - the "father of DNA" himself - recommended a shift in the focus of cancer research from genetics to metabolism.

All that remains for us as a society to say goodbye to the disease of cancer forever is a basic understanding of cellular metabolism, how to address the metabolic dysfunction underlying the disease.

In the next chapter, I will show you exactly how red light works to boost the dysfunctional cellular metabolism underlying cancer and other diseases.

CHAPTER 6

HOW DOES RED LIGHT WORK?

EVERY ONE OF THE ESTIMATED 37.2 trillion cells[1] that make up the human body contain tiny structures within called mitochondria. These organelles are responsible for energy production by the cell, in a process called metabolism.

The following image depicts two healthy mitochondria floating inside a mammalian lung cell, photographed via a transmission electron microscope.

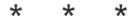

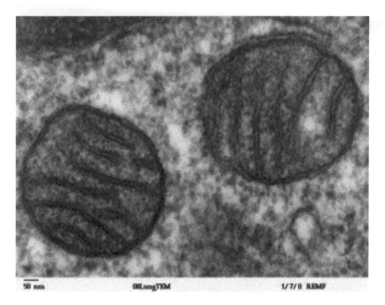

50 nm   ORLungTEM   1/7/0 KEMF

**Two healthy mitochondria floating inside a
mammalian lung cell.**

When a cell is given everything it needs to metabolize
properly – a process involving the chemical oxidation of
glucose into carbon dioxide within the mitochondria – the
cell is healthy. It is the breakdown of efficient metabolism
within cells and tissues that heralds cancer and other
diseases in the body.

Nearly every disease state known to man has been
linked to low mitochondrial activity. Understanding which
foods and factors enhance metabolism, and which inhibit
it are paramount for successfully preventing or reversing
disease.

LOWERING METABOLISM WITH ENVIRONMENTAL TOXINS

One important thing to understand about cellular metabolism is that every step of the process is catalyzed by a specific *enzyme*.

One such enzyme is called cytochrome c oxidase, which was discovered in 1926 by Dr. Otto Warburg, who went on to receive a Nobel Prize for his discovery.[2] This enzyme is critical for oxygen use by cells because it interacts directly with oxygen[3] and catalyzes the very last step in the process of metabolism (called oxidative phosphorylation).[4-5]

Dr. Warburg found that simply by inhibiting cytochrome c oxidase, a healthy cell could be turned into a cancer cell – a finding which has been validated by a number of recent experiments. "Defects in cytochrome c oxidase expression induce a metabolic shift to glycolysis and carcinogenesis," wrote scientists from the University of Pennsylvania in 2015.[6]

A number of chemical toxins have been shown to inhibit cytochrome c oxidase activity, including chemotherapy,[7] cyanide,[8-10] carbon monoxide,[11-12] aluminum phosphide,[13] estrogen,[14] serotonin,[15] endotoxin,[16-17] aflatoxin B1,[18] UVB radiation,[19] X-ray radiation,[20-21] and unsaturated fatty acids.[22]

Here's how it works:

Upon exposure to any of the environmental contaminants listed above, cells produce a free radical called nitric oxide, which binds directly to cytochrome c oxidase, deactivating it.[23-25] For as long as nitric oxide is bound to this enzyme, the cell will have a defective 'cancer' metabolism.

ENHANCING METABOLISM WITH RED LIGHT

The impacts of red and near-infrared light on cellular metabolism are fascinating and unique.

Remarkably, red and near-infrared light have both been proven to actually unbind (aka photodissociate) nitric oxide from the cytochrome c oxidase enzyme,[26-27] restoring its activity. But the truth is even more incredible.

Cytochrome c oxidase is unique in that it actually absorbs light specifically within the red and near-infrared portions of the spectrum. So not only does red and near-infrared light liberate the cytochrome c oxidase enzyme from inhibition by nitric oxide, it also directly energizes this enzyme, which supercharges its activity[28-46]

The result is enhanced cellular metabolism[47-50] and the cascade of beneficial physiological effects that emerge from increased metabolic activity, including:

- Increased energy (ATP) production[49-50]

- Increased cellular oxygenation[52-54]

- Increased blood flow in the body[55-56]

- Increased CO2 production[51]

- Reduced stress hormones[57]

- Reduced lactic acid[49-51]

- Reduced inflammation[58]

- Reduced free radicals[59-64]

It's this cascade of beneficial physiological that can account for most, if not all, of the broad ranging beneficial effects of near-infrared and red light therapies.

Summary:

Red and near-infrared light penetrate deeply into body tissues, where they impart their benefits by enhancing mitochondrial energy production.

CHAPTER 7

IS IT SAFE?

MAINSTREAM DRUG AND SURGICAL-BASED treatments routinely come with massive lists of potentially fatal consequences. Side effects, which are often worse than the conditions being treated, hardly make the medication worth taking. Despite these, most people won't hesitate to take what their doctor prescribes – a fact that never ceases to amaze me.

We live in a culture where people are afraid to drink nourishing raw milk, but won't hesitate to drink diet soda, which contains the insidious poison aspartame.

It would benefit us all if we could come up with some therapies that don't damage us in the process of healing.

How safe is red light therapy?

Of the 50,000+ studies published on red light therapy to date, no adverse side effects have been reported. One of the reasons for this is that the energy intensity of the red and near-infrared wavelengths is extremely low. The amount of energy exposure during red light therapy is so low, in fact, that tissue temperatures don't increase more than a few tenths of a degree. Due to these minute increases in tissue temperature, red light therapy poses no risk of thermal injury.[2]

The virtually non-thermal effects of red light make it particularly attractive for use on fresh injuries when heat would likely worsen swelling and inflammation. Immediate use of red light therapy following an injury is a great strategy to help the body heal itself more rapidly and completely. It can also prevent excessive inflammation that could otherwise exacerbate the injury.

Longtime red light researcher and Harvard scientist Michael Hamblin had this to say about the safety of red light therapy: "In terms of side effects, there are very few side effects. I've occasionally heard of people who put light on their head - I think one person had a headache and a few people felt excessively sleepy."[1]

A number of people have shared with me their miraculous results after using a very small red light therapy device. When it comes to red light therapy, a little bit really does go a long way! (You can read all of their testimonials later in this book). Red or near-infrared light therapy devices emitting as little as 12 watts of light from red and near-infrared LEDs can have remarkably potent effects.

I'm not going to pretend that the FDA-approval stamp is the gold standard for something being safe and effective. There is no shortage of examples where the FDA has passed products or diagnostic tests that it probably shouldn't have; products and tests that weren't effective or even known to be dangerous. So for what it's worth, red light therapy is an FDA-approved treatment for a number of ailments including acne, muscle and joint pain, arthritis, compromised blood circulation, and for reversing hair loss.

PART II

THE PRACTICAL

CHAPTER 8

WHERE TO RECEIVE RED LIGHT THERAPY

TODAY THERE ARE MANY PLACES you can receive red light therapy. Depending on where you live, red light therapy could be available at your local dermatologist, medical spa, day spa, hair salon, tanning salon, physiotherapist and even at your local gym.

Red light therapy administered in a professional setting such as these can be a luxurious experience. In January 2018, I received red laser therapy at a physiotherapist for a knee injury. My overall experience was pleasant and effective but the downside was that it was localized only to my injured knee which means I didn't receive light to my entire body like I had hoped.

Many of the places offering red light therapy mentioned above use full body machines that you either stand or lay down inside. The standing machines require you to stand for the duration of the session and the red light therapy beds are similar to a tanning bed where you lay down inside.

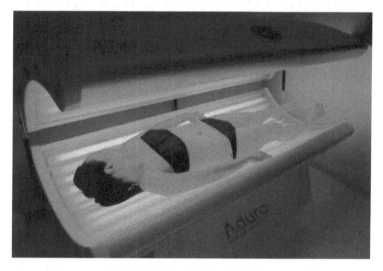

A full-body red light therapy bed

A couple of years ago I received full body red light therapy at a local tanning salon which was essentially a tanning bed except the fluorescent tube lights emitted red radiation instead of UV radiation. When I asked the employees of the salon which wavelengths of red or near-infrared light the bulbs emitted, none could answer my question. I suspect these bulbs emit a wide range of red and/or near-infrared radiation wavelengths, which is good but not as precise as you can be with lasers or LEDs of a single wavelength.

Most full body light therapy machines available today utilize fluorescent bulbs, which are effective, but these bulbs have a number of downsides that retract from their overall benefit.

THE DOWNSIDES OF FLUORESCENT TUBE LIGHTS

Red light therapy administered in a professional setting is excellent because it can save time and will sometimes apply light to your entire body in a single session. However, there are some potential downsides of red light therapy administered with fluorescent tube lights that people need to be aware of.

The first downside is the health risks associated with the fluorescent bulbs themselves.

RADIO FREQUENCY EMISSIONS

Fluorescent bulbs emit radio frequencies. Radio frequencies are the same wireless radiation emitted by cell phones, routers, cordless phones, baby monitors and cell phone towers. Red light radiation and radio frequency radiation have virtually opposite effects on the metabolism of cells. In high enough doses radio frequencies can promote cancer.

While red light boosts cellular metabolism by heightening the activity of the cytochrome c oxidase enzyme, radio frequencies lower metabolism by inhibiting the same enzyme.

ELECTROMAGNETIC FIELDS

In addition to the radio frequency radiation emitted by the fluorescent light bulbs inside a red light therapy machine, the machine itself will emit other harmful factors: electromagnetic fields (EMF).

The two types of electromagnetic fields we are concerned with are electric fields and magnetic fields. Most electronic devices will emit a fairly high amount of electric and magnetic fields, and the more power a device consumes the greater the fields. These fields tend to dissipate over distance, but standing or laying directly inside a red light therapy machine will likely yield a significant dose.

All electronic devices will emit some EMF, and a full body red light therapy bed is no exception. However, red light is so therapeutic that despite radio frequency and EMF emissions, a red light therapy bed will still probably be of great benefit. Radio frequencies and electromagnetic fields tend to retract slightly from that benefit.

A fairly accurate and inexpensive device that can be used to measure the electric and magnetic field emissions from a red light therapy bed or any other electronic device is called a Trifield Meter.©

BE PREPARED TO PAY A PRETTY PENNY

The third and final disadvantage of receiving red light therapy in a professional setting is the price. If you want to receive red light therapy at a local gym or day spa, be prepared to pay a pretty penny, and keep paying for it, because many consecutive sessionss are required to achieve results. Once results have been achieved, additional sessions will be needed to maintain them.

The good news is that the same (or better) results can be obtained from the comfort of your own home at a fraction of the cost.

RED LIGHT THERAPY AT HOME

When the restorative properties of red light were first discovered, LEDs didn't exist; scientists were using red lasers. Lasers devices admitting red or near-infrared light can be purchased, but they cost thousands of dollars, which for most people is not an option.

However, with the invention of LED technology and the subsequent red light therapy devices that are produced using them, suddenly red light therapy became affordable for most people to purchase and use from the comfort of their own homes.

There are many companies selling red light therapy devices online. When I first discovered red light therapy a number of years ago, I purchased two devices from RedLightMan© and put them to the test. Not only were the devices effective, but it was clear that they were built to last. One time I accidentally kicked my larger device off the couch and onto the hard tiled floor below – a 2 foot drop - and surprisingly it didn't cause any damage to the device and it still works to this day.

A well-built product that changes people's lives by improving their health is one I can get behind, so I decided to produce my own exclusive line of red light therapy devices for my EndAllDisease online store. Like I said, there are many places online you can get red light therapy devices but these are the devices I use and recommend.

To give you an example of what high quality red light therapy devices look like, check out our lights at EndAllDisease.com/store.

Conclusion

As you've seen in this chapter, there are many ways to receive red light therapy, with varying devices and costs associated with each method.

All red light machines have their own set of advantages and disadvantages. It's important to experiment until you find what works best for you.

At the end of the day, nothing is better than owning your own personal red and near-infrared light therapy device made with high quality LEDs. Buying your own device and using it from the comfort of your own home will give you all the benefits of expensive laser therapy sessions in clinical settings, while saving you hundreds, if not thousands of dollars in the process.

CHAPTER 9

YOUR COMPLETE GUIDE TO RED LIGHT THERAPY AT HOME

AS SOMEONE WHO HAS BEEN researching and experimenting with red light therapy for over 6 years, I have learned a number of things about what works and what doesn't. I've helped hundreds of people develop specific light therapy protocols and the feedback I've received has been invaluable. It is from this collection of experiences that I share my most important concepts and strategies that will allow you to achieve the greatest possible results from red light therapy.

On the surface, red light therapy is simple: Switch on your light, aim it at the body part you wish to help, and then shine it there for 10-20 minutes. However, there are a number of important factors that need to be considered to get the best possible results. These considerations can be the difference between remarkable healing and no healing.

SIMPLICITY IS THE KEY TO SUCCESS

One of the most important factors for success with red light therapy is consistency. In order to remain consistent, each session must be made as simple as possible and the results must be noticeable. The purpose of this chapter is to help you make your red light therapy sessions as easy and effective as possible. If using the device isn't simple and the results are not noticeable, then it's only a matter of time before your device will sit in a corner collecting dust.

A good example of what *not* to do comes from a friend of mine who was using red light to restore hair growth on the top of his head. For his first session, he sat down and applied the light to the skin on top of his head by holding the device there for the entire session. As you might expect, the most noticeable results he got were sore shoulders! After realizing this was an uncomfortable way to administer the light, he tried a different approach. His strategy this time was to attach the red light device to the inside of a lampshade and wear that on his head. This story confirmed to me that more practical information was needed on exactly how to administer red light therapy.

Inspired by this and other stories, I present to you the 6 most important factors to consider when designing your red light protocol.

1. Creating a Space for Light Therapy

2. Body position

3. Light position

4. Light distance

5. Session frequency

6. Session duration

1. CREATE A SPACE FOR LIGHT THERAPY

If for each red light therapy session you had to carry your light up 3 flights of stairs, every step coated in hot, gummy tar with 5 inch nails sticking straight up out of some of them like in the movie *Home Alone,* then plug your device into the wall and lay down on a cold, hard cement floor naked for 15 minutes while you apply the light - how many times would you *actually* do it before quitting?

This extreme example I think most vividly illustrates my point: If your red light therapy sessions are not simple and pleasurable, you will not do them consistently for a long period of time. Instead, you will probably do it a few times and then quit.

Intentionally creating a space dedicated to red light therapy is important for your success. Your light therapy space must make your sessions both simple and pleasurable. This space could include a towel, blanket or yoga mat spread out on the floor where you can sit or lay down. A pillow or two can also be a good addition. If you plan to use a timer other than your phone, keep this in your light therapy space. Locating your space near a power outlet and having your light plugged into it at all times so it's ready for use is also important for simplicity. And of course, adding to your space anything else that you feel will help you focus and relax completely can also be helpful.

In the past I have tried keeping a device beside my bed, with the intent of using my bed for light therapy sessions. This may sound like the ideal location for red light therapy because it's simple and extremely comfortable but I've found it to not be ideal. In fact, it may be the extreme comfort itself that is its biggest downfall. Most of us associate a bed with sleeping - and given the fact that the best times for light therapy sessions are morning and night, you may find that it's much easier to just fall asleep rather than set a timer and *put on the red light*.

Create a comfortable space that will make your red light therapy sessions as simple as possible.

2. BODY POSITION

The way you position your body during red light therapy sessions is the next important factor to consider. If your body is positioned in a way that is uncomfortable and doesn't allow you to fully relax, then it's only a matter of time before you lose interest and stop using the device.

In life, people tend to be greater motivated to avoid things that are unpleasant rather than to engage in things that are pleasant and rewarding. This is why it is essential to position your body in a way that is entirely comfortable and allows your body to relax completely.

The three basic options for body position include standing, sitting and laying down.

BODY POSITION: STANDING

Some red light therapy devices on the market today are designed to have the person stand up for the entire session. These include long rectangular LED light panels which are held upright by a stand or mounted on the wall, and also some futuristic-looking, standing vertical light therapy booths with a swinging door for entry and exit.

The concept of standing during light therapy seems great in theory, *but who wants to stand in one spot twice a day for 15-20 minutes in a row!?* Standing in one spot for long periods of time can be very uncomfortable, as a constant contraction of many muscles is required in order to support the weight of your body. This means that standing up during light therapy makes fully-relaxing impossible. Furthermore, many people quickly feel soreness or pain in their feet, knees, hips while standing in one place. This pain can just compound the discomfort of having to stand for 20 minutes in a row.

There is one final disadvantage of standing: The more your body is deficient in red light, the more you are likely to fall asleep during red light therapy. This means that by standing, you're missing out on one of the most beautiful parts about light therapy. I don't think I could fall asleep while standing if I tried, but if it happened it could be a dangerous situation. Imagine falling asleep while standing up and collapsing to the floor like a sack of potatoes.

Due to the many disadvantages of standing during light therapy, you will probably not continue therapy consistently and over the long term. However, keep in mind everybody is different and you may not feel the way I do about it. Overall, shining the light on your skin is *far* more important than dwelling endlessly on body position.

BODY POSITION: SITTING

A seated body position during red light therapy can be fitting for some people, particularly if you're able to sit in a comfortable recliner. A comfortable recliner or even a sofa affords a safe space in which you can relax. These are the main advantages of sitting, but sitting comes not without its own set of things to consider.

The main downsides of the seated position are as follows:

- Sitting requires supportive muscles to contract, preventing complete relaxation

- Sitting makes it difficult to properly position your red light

- Sitting can be uncomfortable or even painful for some people

Similar to the standing position, sitting requires your body to contract a number of supportive muscles for the entire session. Any muscles that aren't permitted to relax fully will prevent you from receiving maximum benefit from red light therapy.

Sitting also makes it difficult to effectively position your red light. For example, if you wanted to put your light directly against your forehead to boost brain function, regulate emotions, reduce anxiety and depression, detoxify the brain and boost cognitive function, it would be difficult to do that while seated. The only way I can think of to make that happen would be to hold the device the entire time, which is highly inconvenient and uncomfortable. If you choose to sit during red light therapy sessions, set the device down to avoid having to hold it the entire time. We will talk more about light position shortly, but for now it's important to note that the seated position makes it difficult to find a spot for your light that is close to your skin.

Lastly, for some people sitting can be uncomfortable or even painful. Many people spend 40 or more hours a week sitting while driving to work and then sitting while at work. As a culture we tend to sit far too much. Sitting seems to be okay for brief periods of time, but the evidence shows too much can be detrimental to health. It can inhibit blood circulation, reduce flexibility and even cause back pain for many people. For those who already sit too much, it's probably best to avoid the seated position during red light therapy sessions.

BODY POSITION: LAYING DOWN

Laying down is *the gold standard* for red light therapy. It is comfortable, it allows you to relax every muscle in your body, and it is the only position that is entirely safe for you to fall asleep in.

In many dermatologist offices where red light therapy is offered, light therapy devices are hung from the ceiling and patients are put on massage therapy tables unclothed beneath the light. Finding an above supportive structure upon which you can hang your light may require a bit of creativity and engineering, but if you can manage it's an excellent accomplishment because now you've created a solid, permanent, and comfortable space.

Currently I use red light therapy while laying on a yoga mat that I've placed on the floor with a couple of pillows for added comfort. I've got the light plugged into the wall so it can be turned on with the flick of a switch.

Creating a space which allows you to lay down during red light therapy sessions is the best way to do it from home. Your therapy space can range from very simple, like mine, to a more complex clinical-like setting. I recommend laying down during red light therapy, and also encourage you to experiment with body positions to find out what works best for you.

3. LIGHT POSITION

In this section, I'll talk primarily about where and how to position your light while laying down during red light therapy. But first, a few quick words about how you can position your light while standing or sitting.

LIGHT POSITION WHILE STANDING

While standing, the position of your light can be either on a vertical stand or mounted to a wall. This is advantageous because you don't have to hold the light the entire time, but not ideal because you have to actually stand for the entire session as previously discussed.

LIGHT POSITION WHILE SITTING

While sitting, the two best options for light location are on a table in front of you or on your lap facing you. However, these methods also come with some obvious disadvantages. These light positions make it difficult to apply light anywhere but your stomach or a portion of your upper body and face from a distance.

LIGHT POSITION WHILE LAYING DOWN

Compared to standing or sitting, positioning your light while laying down is a breeze. All you have to do is lay down, then place the light down beside you on the floor or bed aimed at the body part you wish to apply the light.

Got a sore knee? No problem. Lay down, then lay the light down in front of you on the ground against your knee, set the timer, and relax.

Got pain in your lower back? No problem. Lay down, then lay the light down behind you directed at the area that is causing you pain, set the timer, and relax.

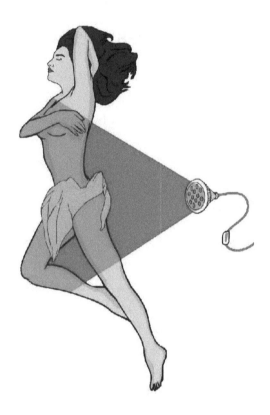

Want to do a whole body session? No problem. Lay down, then lay the light down a foot in front of you - aimed at the middle of your torso while in the fetal position – so the light hits every inch of skin from your upper legs, stomach, chest and upper arms, then set the timer, and relax.

Laying down is the ideal body position during red light therapy. It affords you comfortability and safety while simplifying light position and eliminating the need to hold the light for the entire session. It's this simplicity in combination with your ability to relax in this position that will provide maximum results and make you excited for your next session.

4. LIGHT DISTANCE

Light distance refers to the distance you place the light from your body during red light therapy. As you move the red light farther away from your body, two things happen:

1. The light will spread out and reach more cells simultaneously

2. Less photons of light will reach each individual cell (since they will be spread out amongst many more cells)

Since a light farther away from the body will reach more cells, positioning the light 1-3 feet away can be helpful for full body therapy. However, it's important to understand that less light photons will reach each cell at a distance, which means your session time will need to be increased in order for cells to receive the same dose as they would if the light was closer to your body. The ideal in this case might be 20-30 minutes as opposed to 12 minutes.

If you want to reach tissues deep within the body, like a knee injury, for example, put the light directly up against the skin of your knee. This will allow a concentrated dose of light to penetrate deeply and reach all tissues within your knee joint. With the light directly against your skin, less time will be needed to fully saturate your knee cells with a healthy dose of red light. 12-15 minutes should be plenty of time.

For all practical purposes, that's virtually everything you need to know regarding light positioning. For those looking for more highly technical information on red light dosing, sign up for my newsletter on EndAllDisease.com and receive my free Red Light Therapy Dose Guide.

5. SESSION DURATION

Session duration can be defined as the number of minutes light is exposed to the body during a single red light therapy session. Through experimentation with various session times, I have gathered some wisdom which I will share with you in this section.

Although some science has been done on trying to determine the optimal session times for various conditions, keep in mind that nothing is set in stone. I always encourage people to do their own experimentation and see how different session lengths make you feel.

For your first ever light therapy session, I recommend a full body session for about 20 minutes. Simply lay in the fetal position, fully unclothed, with the light facing your stomach and chest. Your goal will be to reach as many cells as possible. From this position is should be possible to reach your upper legs, stomach, chest and upper arms all in one shot.

If you bought a red light specifically for an injured ankle or pain in a specific part of your body, perform two sessions daily – one full-body and the other directly at the site of pain or injury.

My own experience has helped me narrow down what I believe to be *my own* optimal session time. For me, 15 minute sessions – with the light directly against my body - are good. It's an amount of time that isn't so long that I end up counting the seconds for it to end.

Don't take my word for it though. Experiment with various session times – 10 minutes, 15 minutes, 20 minutes, all the way up to 2 hours (if you have a light with a cooling fan) - to find your optimal session time. Simply set the timer on your phone, switch on your light, then lay back and enjoy.

6. SESSION FREQUENCY

Session frequency can be defined as the number of sessions you undergo each day. As a general guideline, studies have demonstrated that somewhere between 2 and 20 red light therapy sessions per week are effective. That's 2-3 times per day. However, there should be no qualms about using your device more if you want to do some experimentation of your own, as red light therapy is remarkably safe.

In my own experience, two sessions per day have been very effective and that's what is probably best for most people with health problems. I recommend one session first thing in the morning and another at night before bed. In the morning, red light therapy will energize you and prepare you for your day, and red light at night will alleviate any stress you may have accumulated that day, allowing you to fully relax into a peaceful, deep, restful sleep.

Since red light energizes cells within the body, some people have asked if it can interrupt their sleep. From my experience, red light can actually *improve* sleep quality by reducing the levels of cortisol and adrenaline in your body. Reducing stress hormones will increase efficient energy production by cells - and a well-energized cell is a relaxed cell. Red light therapy before bed is one of the best ways to improve sleep quality.

As always, I encourage you to do your own experimentation to find your optimal session frequency. You've got everything to gain and nothing to lose.

CHAPTER 10

THE #1 BIGGEST MISTAKE PEOPLE MAKING DURING RED LIGHT THERAPY

SOME PEOPLE HAVE COME TO me for advice, frustrated from the lack of success they'd been having with red light therapy. I asked them to describe their routines to me and found a number of mistakes they were making. One mistake in particular was common among almost everybody who hadn't been getting results. After making just one simple change to their protocols, their limited successes were transformed into profound results almost every time.

In this chapter I will teach you the #1 biggest mistake people during red light therapy so you can save time by learning from other people's mistakes rather than learning the hard way. With the right information and a few simple adjustments, frustrations and lack of success can be converted into remarkable results.

The following case study is probably the best way to illustrate for you what a good light therapy protocol looks like. The principles gained from this experience in the story can help you create your own successful protocol for whatever ails you. At the end of this chapter I will present the one single thing you can do to accelerate your success more than anything else.

CASE STUDY: ARTHRITIS IN HAND

A woman came to me with pain and inflammation in her hand, which had been officially diagnosed as arthritis by her doctor. Treatment by her doctor failed and came with many unwanted side effects, so she began trying red light therapy, but up until that point wasn't having any success. In the interest of keeping her name anonymous I will call her Jane.

I asked Jane how she had been positioning herself - standing, seated or laying down? In a seated position, Jane replied, with her hand flat on the table in front of her and the light suspended from a hook above and pointing directly downwards. She had done a few sessions a week for about 12 minutes each session, but it wasn't relieving her pain and inflammation.

My job at this point was to give Jane some advice on how she could have greater success and eliminate the pain and immobility in her hand. While the impact of diet on the genesis and on alleviating such a condition I think is probably more important than the red light itself, I didn't give her any nutrition advice. However, I never leave a stone unturned for my readers, so I'm going to quickly summarize my thoughts on the relationship between nutrition and arthritis for you now.

Dietary Changes for Arthritis

Based on my research, the most significant dietary factor causing both pain and inflammation in the body are the consumption of polyunsaturated fatty acids (PUFA). In my book *Cancer: The Metabolic Disease Unravelled*, I present a mountain of evidence revealing the following negative health consequences of PUFA:

- It directly inhibits the cytochrome c oxidase enzyme
- It inhibits the immune system by shrinking the thymus gland and by directly killing white blood cells
- It lowers oxygen use by cells
- It inhibits thyroid function in at least five ways

It's the slow and gradual accumulation of PUFA within the tissues of the body over a lifetime of consuming foods containing them that overwhelms the body's ability to switch off stress/inflammation.

Based on this research, my practical advice is to *increase the
ratio* of saturated to polyunsaturated fatty acids in your
diet. This dietary modification is paramount for any kind
of permanent resolution of arthritis.

Polyunsaturated fatty acids include any oils which are
liquid at room temperature. Olive oil and Avocado oil are
lower in PUFA than corn oil, fish oil and other nut and
seed oils, but the safest of fats are the most highly
saturated fats including coconut oil, butter, chocolate fat,
beef and lamb fat.

MODIFICATIONS TO JANE'S RED LIGHT THERAPY PROTOCOL

It's important to understand that although the chronic
pain Jane had been experiencing was localized to her hand,
arthritis is a whole-body systemic condition, not a local
issue. In other words, it wasn't a defect in her hand that
was causing the problem, but rather the overall condition
of her body. In arthritis, the body is unable to heal from
damaged tissue and the ideal strategy should include red
light applied directly to the affected tissue as well as the
entire body.

I gave Jane some practical advice on how she could
improve her approach. Instead of aiming the red light
solely at her hand rested on a table, I recommended that
she try to reach as many cells as possible during her
sessions, using the following suggestions:

- Remove all clothing

- Lay down on your side in a comfortable place in the fetal position

- Place your red light 1 foot away on the bed/ground, facing your diaphragm (midway between your stomach and chest)

- Rest your arthritic hand directly against your stomach

With this approach, not only will the red light boost the metabolism of cells in her hand, but the light will do the same - inches deep into her body – in every cell from her knees to her stomach to her chest to her upper arms. Not surprisingly, after applying her new protocol Jane's results have been profound – *even without any dietary changes.* With consistent red light therapy sessions every morning and night, mobility returned to her hands and the painful swelling and inflammation has resided.

Mechanism of Action

For those interested in the mechanism of action, the key reason for this is the inhibition of the enzyme COX-2 by red light. This enzyme is responsible for the release of free fatty acids (PUFA) from cells (a process called lipolysis). By inhibiting lipolysis, the constant release of toxic PUFA in the damaged area is 'switched off'.

For permanent resolution of arthritis, as previously stated, replacing toxic unsaturated fats in the diet with protective, saturated fats will also be necessary.

The #1 Most Powerful Strategy for Success

THE #1 BIGGEST MISTAKE PEOPLE MAKE DURING TREATMENT

Reaching as many cells as possible during red light therapy is the most important principle to apply to your protocol. By maximizing the number of cells which receive red light, the amount of ATP and healing carbon dioxide produced metabolically are increased, which benefits all cells and systems of the body.

The best way to nourish the body both systemically and locally is to do two red light therapy sessions per day – one in the morning and one at night. In the morning, shine light on your whole body and at night, shine light on the local area that's causing symptoms. Continue with this regimen consistently for a week or more and take note of any progress.

Applying red light to a localized area where you are experiencing symptoms is important for relieving those symptoms, but reaching as many cells, tissues and organs within the body with red light as possible through full-body therapy sessions is the most powerful strategy for success.

CHAPTER 11

REMARKABLE SUCCESS STORIES

SINCE PUBLISHING THIS BOOK I have received a number of exciting testimonials from people who have had incredible results using red light therapy. Most of these people had tried various mainstream and alternative therapies with no success. Time and time again, red light therapy has succeeded where other therapies have failed. In this chapter I will share with you a few of these testimonials.

SUCCESS STORIES 1&2: SHOULDER PAIN ELIMINATED WITH RED LIGHT

A shoulder injury is a debilitating condition that can affect every aspect of your life – from work to leisure to sleep and everything in between. Shoulder injuries can occur while playing sports, during exercise, while at work or during any other strenuous physical activity. The biggest issue with injuries today is that most people never really obtain complete healing and consequently must deal with pain and immobility for the rest of their lives.

Many people resort to surgery for their injuries, which is often completely unnecessary and can make the situation much worse. The following is a brief summary on the subject of unnecessary surgery from my book *The Cancer Industry*:

Unnecessary Surgery

Research on unnecessary surgery began in 1974, after a US congressional report estimated that 2.4 million unnecessary surgeries were performed every year, killing nearly 12,000 patients. This report caught the eye of Harvard professor and former surgeon Lucian Leape, who has been following this line of research ever since.

Leape's take today? "Things haven't changed very much."

A 2016 review of the latest research on unnecessary surgery states, "Worldwide every year millions of patients go under knife, but many of them are enduring great pain and shelling out thousands and dollars for surgeries they don't really need."

Two people have sent me testimonials after using red light for chronic shoulder pain they had been experiencing for many years. Each story is slightly different yet both people ended up having fantastic results. Both stories are presented below.

The first success story is from a friend of mine who had been experiencing shoulder pain for over a decade. She told me there wasn't any one particular incident that caused damage to her shoulder, so the origins of the pain were unknown. However, due to the fact that she sat at a desk for 40+ hours a week at her job, she suspected the pain had to do with her overall lack of movement and exercise in life.

She had tried chiropractor, osteopathy, and acupuncture for her shoulder but nothing relieved her pain. Then she heard about red light therapy and put a red light therapy device to the test. "My pain was gone after the first treatment!," she exclaimed to me the following day. After just one 20 minute session applying red light to her shoulder, her u☐☐ untreatable' shoulder pain that had been troubling her for over 10 years was completely alleviated.

The second shoulder pain success story I received came from a woman who had also been experiencing shoulder pain for many years. "I went to numerous doctors, therapist, healers, I even went to a shaman, no one can explain why, and I lived in quiet agony," she remarked. I'll paste her full testimonial below so you can read it yourself, but the results were so significant that after just 3 days she was actually able to go rock climbing.

"I just want to say thank you, Mark. I've had shoulder pain for years, I went to numerous doctors, therapist, healers, I even went to a shaman, no one can explain why, and I lived in quiet agony. Today marks the 3rd day I'm using the light device purchased from your web store and I'm already feeling a lot better. Full of vitality and good vibes, I even went rock climbing yesterday. Thank you so so so much, blessings to you."

SUCCESS STORY #3: EYESIGHT IMPROVED WITH RED LIGHT

As a society we are conditioned to believe that a decline in visual acuity with age is unavoidable and irreversible. We should all just accept the 'fact' that as we age we will eventually need glasses, right? Evidence is mounting, from both scientific studies and from personal testimony of red light therapy device owners, that red light *can* in fact correct poor vision.

Previously in this book, I presented a study in which elderly people were given red light therapy for their age-related macular degeneration. The study showed that the red light significantly improved the participant's visual acuity, and remarkably, the benefits – from as little as four sessions over a two week period – lasted up to 3 years. However, to date there are no studies that I'm aware of which have tested the ability of red light on the average non-elderly person with suboptimal vision. Thanks to the valuable testimony of a red light therapy device owner, we now have brand new empirical evidence suggesting that red light's vision-boosting benefits are not just for the elderly.

A woman named Kaya from Toronto, Ontario had an eyeglass prescription of 4.5/20 when she discovered red light therapy. She read the study showing red light improved visual acuity in elderly with macular degeneration and decided to test red light therapy on her own eyesight using a red light device. She sent me the following testimony:

"Wonderful!!!! I am recommending this to so many people as the results are so good!!! My eyes are healing almost perfectly...they were 4.5 in prescription and yesterday I went to optometrist and one eye is now perfect 20/20 and the other one is close behind!!!... My Optometrist is super perplexed and I laughed so hard. She said eyes like mine aren't supposed to correct like that!"

If you're interested in using red light therapy for improving your eyesite, the exact protocol that I recommend can be found in the *Bonus Q&A* chapter of this book.

SUCCESS STORY #4: THE CASE OF THE MISSING BONE

This next testimonial comes from an American man named Al Gray and his wife, who both benefitted from a handheld light for their distinctly different health issues. Al used red light on his hernia, and his wife used red light for pain caused by a bone in her thumb which mysteriously went missing and was replaced by a plastic one. Both of these testimonials combined are very unique and fascinating cases of recovery. Up until this point I had never heard of anybody using red light for these conditions so we're breaking new ground with this one. Here's their testimony:

"I was thinking of writing to you and reporting what to me was an amazing experience with the light. I'm going to bypass the survey form and just share my experience.

My True Love woke up one morning sometime in March of this year with a left thumb that was non-functional. She went to the ER and they took an X-ray. The X-ray showed that the bone that connects the thumb to the wrist was completely gone. It was like Scotty from Star Trek had beamed it up. The wrist bone and the thumb bone were just fine. No sign of deterioration on either of them. It was strange to see. If the other bones showed signs of deterioration, it could be explained as osteoporosis. But the bone was just gone.

So she made an appointment with a surgeon in a nearby town and he replaced the missing bone with a plastic bone. Gave her a brace to wear and sent her home. She went back for regular checkups and after a few months was allowed to remove the brace. There was some residual pain that seemed to decrease as time went on. Many weeks

went by and the pain had decreased to the point where the only time it hurt was when she moved her thumb. Not a life-limiting pain, but really annoying.

She used her thumb for something a week or two ago and the pain was constant. She agreed to let me use the red light on the thumb. The pain went away. And miraculously, it has not come back. The thumb is still weak. She has trouble with door knobs and jar lids but she has no pain. To me, that is a miracle.

On a note of personal experience, I have used it on my hernia and the hernia is shrinking. It's shrinking very fast, and when it is finally gone I will send you an e-mail, just in case you can't hear my whoop of joy up in Canada."

- Al Gray

MORE SUCCESS STORIES

Excellent results from red light therapy have been had by many more people who have followed up with me to share their stories. Some of the responses weren't as long and the situations weren't as thoroughly described as the previous ones, but nonetheless they are absolute gems!

It never ceases to amaze me what red light can do for people. And knowing that my work is truly helping alleviate suffering and other problems in people's lives has truly made all the hard work and effort worthwhile. Even if just one person had benefitted from this work it would've made all the hard work worthwhile, and yet it's clear that it has touched the lives of many more.

Here are some more testimonials from people who have benefitted from red light therapy:

"My knees feel so much better. More stable. I'll continue using.
- Linda Redman from Maryland, Age 50-60

"It seems to be healing a fistula on my gums very quickly."
- Richard from the US, Age 30-40

"Helping adult acne and scars; better focus throughout the day and better, more restful sleep at night."
- Haley Wickenheimer from Michigan, Age 20-30

"Greatly reduces pain in knee that has no meniscus, reduces swelling in ankles. Using on different parts of my body as prescribed in your book. Skin on face, chest and arms much improved. Like the warmth, and generally

enjoy using this device."
- Keener Janssen from California, Age 60+

"It has lessened the pain from a sprained ankle so that there is much less pain when I put weight on it."
- Marianna McClymonds from Arizona, Age 60+

"A friend of mine was recently diagnosed with shingles. He has been using red light therapy on the infected area. To date, the shingles have not spread and the itch is minimal. I call it my miracle light! It has helped with my knees and it has helped with his shingles. I use it every day and have been telling everyone about it!"
- Teresa Van Parys from Cambridge, Age 50-60

"I got the handheld light for my Dad, he broke his toe a few weeks before he got the light. It was swollen and killing him, after 2-3 days of shinning on his toe the pain went away and swelling gone amazing. He also fell and hurt his back he could barely move after using the light on his back within 10 minutes the pain was gone unbelievable. I want to wait a few months and see if it will work for his hearing loss, either way, I want to leave a good review on your site. I was a pro cyclist and nordic ski racer, I'm getting back into racing so I'm going to save up and buy the full-body light to help with recovery and endurance. I've watched all your videos already, keep up the good work."
- Mitch

"I got the red light mainly for me, but my nine-year-old son has sensory processing disorder and Dyslexia and I thought that it might help with his anxiety. Bedtime can be a real struggle because by that point of the day he is in sensory overload, and he gets hyperactive and rambunctious (about the time the rest of the family is slowing down). The other night we were having an especially tough time, so I needed to excuse myself to the shower and have a moment to regroup. I was running out of patience and ideas. A few minutes later he came in the bathroom and asked what that big light was in my room. I told him what it was and said he was welcome to lay in front of it for a few minutes. When I came out of the shower, he was a different kid. Like he had just gotten out of a 60 min Swedish massage. He was calm and peaceful, and said "Hi Momma" with a sweet smile. He was able to get in bed and stay still long enough to drift off to sleep. Best $799 I ever spent."

- Jamie Jones

"Skin looks better after only 2 weeks. Dark spots on face are noticeably lighter. My vision is improving!!"

- Susan from Toronto, Age 60+

"Pain in the shoulder has been noticeably reduced. Range of motion is much improved. Should get better with continued use."

- D. Hines from Toronto, Age 40-50

"Reduced pain significantly after heavy physical work-outs. I sleep better as well. Also reduced some of my wrinkles."

- Daniel Mischuk from Toronto, Age 60+

"While I intended to use the red light therapy device for healing hearing loss and helping to reduce the appearance of scars which it has, I have also noticed an additional benefit that I did not expect. I fell asleep while using the device and subsequently had extremely vivid dreams and experienced a very profound deep state of relaxation. I know use my red light therapy device while meditating with fantastic results."

- Adrian Bankhead from Washington, Age 40-50

"I am finding that my nails are growing like crazy and they are very strong. I also feel a bit more refreshed when I wake up in the morning and not as groggy. My purchase was mainly for my thyroid and to regrow hair. I shine it on my full body, thyroid and sometimes on my scalp. I have been using this 1x a day for almost a month."

Remi from Boise, Idaho, Age 40-50

"1) I have an unstable arthritic knee with major cartilage loss. After 3 weeks of red light therapy on the knee it has stabilized and the pain is greatly reduced. I no longer limp. 2) I use it on my torso as instructed and am feeling stronger and more alert generally. I am losing belly fat."

- Harold F Hees from Forth Worth, Texas, Age 60+

"So far incredible pain relief, anxiety relief, enhanced sleep, better digestion, weight loss(7lbs), wound healing really fast, greater sense of wellbeing, rash clearing."

- Barbara Malamatenios from California, Age 60+

"Far surpassed my expectations! My facial skin is literally glowing as a result of five minutes daily exposure to the red light. Larger areas (thighs, stomach, breasts) are also responding nicely. More time is needed to achieve the overall result I'm searching for in these areas, but I never would have thought I'd see this kind of reversal to the damage that results from pregnancy and breast feeding. I won't be needing plastic surgery and I am absolutely overjoyed that my greatest joy (being a mother) hasn't cost me my figure after all."

- Samantha Brown from Florida, Age 40-50

"So far a cut finger, in 20 minutes closed up. I could not believe my eyes. I held it for 20 minutes in a tissue, the bleeding continued, then I remembered my Red light therapy lamp and viola...right before my eyes it was healed! The deep cut from a very sharp knife almost seemed instantly and it was gone! Also, my lower back feels great. The varicose veins on my right leg have almost disappeared! It fascinates me to witness these miracles!!

- Dianne from Peterborough, Ontario, Age 60+

"I suffer from Complex Regional Syndrome in my right arm and hand that I injured in a fall after work 12 years ago and now have nerve damage, always have pain. Once you injure yourself it can move, as I rolled my ankle last year has now moved to my foot as well as my hand so my whole right side is in pain... During the week I use this [a red light therapy device] for 20 minutes each morning and it's helping me be able to use my arm a lot better. I have the weekends off. And once the weekend ends I use it again during the week and feel a benefit for a better quality of life. I'm looking forward to the next few months as most things take a few months before you see the real benefits. All I can say is thank you Mark for all your information to help people like myself."

- Debbie from Australia, Age 50-60

If you have a red light therapy success story that you'd like to share, I've created a form that I'm using to collect more case studies that could be featured in upcoming videos, articles and maybe even in this book.

To share your red light success story, go to https://endalldisease.com/redlightsuccess

CHAPTER 12

MY EXPERIENCE WITH RED LIGHT THERAPY

I FIRST LEARNED ABOUT RED light therapy in 2014 while searching online for effective alternative treatments that I could use to improve my health and life. At that point I had tried dozens of other supplements and foods with various successes and red light sounded promising so I decided to put it to the test.

I purchased a red and near-infrared light device and the effects were potent and almost immediate. After 12 minutes of shining the light on my stomach and chest area, I felt noticeably more relaxed - as if a weight had been lifted off my chest.

Next, I held the light up against my forehead to see how red light would impact my brain function. I didn't notice anything until I left home and began interacting with people. The effects were profound. My brain cells felt energized and the quality and speed of my thoughts and speech were markedly enhanced.

Today I use red light twice a day – once in the morning and once at night - on my brain and body. On my brain I use it to ensure my cognition is at peak function throughout the day. With full-body therapy I ensure the light reaches as many cells as possible, including my thyroid, which enhances metabolism and energy levels throughout the day. I also ensure the light reaches my testicles, which provides a noticeable enhancement in energy and sexual function.

In addition to owning and using my own red light devices at home, I've also tried red light therapy at a local tanning salon. The machine they offered was basically a tanning bed equipped with pink fluorescent tube lights.

The effects of red light therapy in a tanning bed didn't feel as pronounced as using my own personal LED light therapy devices. I suspect this had to do with the fact that fluorescent lights emit radio frequency radiation, which detracts from the beneficial effects of red light. Also, the employee at the salon couldn't tell me specifically the wavelength or wavelengths of light the machine was emitting, so the difference could also have to do with wavelength. Another downside of receiving red light therapy at a salon or dermatologist office is the price. Sometimes these places charge as much as $50-$100 for a single session.

It is far cheaper and more convenient to buy your own device and reap the benefits of light therapy at home. The high-quality red and near-infrared light therapy devices available on EndAllDisease.com are manufactured with LEDs rated to last up to 50,000 hours, which means purchasing a single device could last a lifetime. These are the devices I use myself and recommend.

Red and near-infrared light therapies have provided me with enormous benefit and I want to help others find the same healing. I use and will continue to use red light therapy devices on a daily basis probably for the rest of my life.

CHAPTER 13

TWO PROVEN WAYS TO ACCELERATE HEALING

BY NOW YOU UNDERSTAND THAT red light therapy is remarkably safe and effective. But no matter how remarkable something may be, it can always be better. In this bonus chapter, I will give you two scientifically proven healing strategies that can be used in conjunction with red light therapy. When combined, these strategies will synergistically enhance the effectiveness of red light.

The two healing strategies involve applying certain substances to the area just prior to applying red light. When combined, a synergy is achieved, meaning the total effect from both therapies together is greater than the sum of each individual therapy.

HONEY

Honey has long been known for its powerful antibiotic effects. Since ancient times it has been used for superficial wounds such as burns, scrapes or cuts. Today the remarkable disinfectant ability of honey has been validated by scientific research.

In the past, the exact property of honey that exhibited the antibacterial effects was not known, but today it has been established: hydrogen peroxide ($H2O2$). It's interesting to note that the hydrogen peroxide content in natural honeys can vary as much as 100-fold from one honey to the next. Honey is also antibacterial because it is "hygroscopic, which means that it can draw moisture out of the environment and dehydrate bacteria, and its high sugar content and low pH can also prevent the microbes from growth."[1] One study found that applying honey dressings to burn wounds can outperform mainstream ointment silver sulfadiazine.[2]

In 2018, some forward-thinking scientists from Delhi tested the effects of honey and red light therapy on burn wounds in rats. One group of rats received red light therapy only, and the other group of rats received red light therapy after honey was applied directly to their wound. The study found that the wounds of rats nourished with red light and honey caused less pain and healed more quickly than the wounds of rats that received red light alone. "Thus, the findings of present study signify that the combination of medicinal honey and PBMT accelerates the repair process of burn wounds," they concluded.[3]

The increased healing triggered by the honey can be partially attributed to its antiseptic properties, but more fundamentally, applying honey to damaged cells provides them with a virtually unlimited supply of the essential nutrient glucose. This glucose abundance allows cells to produce as much ATP and CO_2 as needed to orchestrate rapid and complete healing. Wounds packed with honey are likely to heal quickly and scarlessly. Consuming honey orally before sessions is also highly recommended for this same reason.

When you are wounded, remember to apply honey directly to the injured tissue, consume some honey orally and then *put on the red light*.

COCONUT OIL

For those who don't have access to honey or find it too sticky and unpleasant to work with, I present to you an alternative that can provide similar synergistic benefits when used with red light.

Coconut oil is a potent antibiotic that can be used topically and consumed orally to accelerate the healing of wounds. Based on research from the coconut oil chapter I wrote in my book *Cancer: The Metabolic Disease Unravelled*, the numerous properties of coconut oil for healing are discussed below.

First, coconut oil has potent antibacterial,[4-5] antifungal[6-7] and antiviral[8-9] properties. This makes it another good selection as a topical ointment for wounds. When consumed orally, coconut oil can also help eliminate any internal fungal, bacterial and viral assailants that may be inhibiting the healing process.

By applying coconut oil topically, damaged tissues are afforded an abundance of easily-utilizable saturated free fatty acids that can be used to restore efficient metabolism. Scientific studies have demonstrated, much like honey, that coconut oil applied topically to wounds can accelerate the healing process.[10-11]

Honey and coconut oil are two useful adjuncts to red light therapy which can be used both topically and orally to synergistically enhance the already potent effects of red light.

CHAPTER 14

YOUR QUESTIONS ANSWERED

SINCE PUBLISHING THIS BOOK I have received numerous emails from customers and fans asking various questions about red and near-infrared light therapy. I decided to answer a number of the most common and interesting questions in this chapter.

"DO I NEED TO WEAR EYE PROTECTION DURING RED LIGHT THERAPY?"

To date, no eye damage has ever been reported from red or near-infrared light therapies. And to the contrary, red light has been found to actually improve visual acuity in some cases. So like all cells of the human body, eyes kept open and uncovered will likely obtain benefit from the light.

If your light is just too bright for you to keep your eyes open during red light therapy, then go ahead and close your eyes. The light will still be able to penetrate your eye lids and reach the cells of your eyes during sessions. If it's still too bright, then by all means, put on some goggles.

"WHAT IS A WAVELENGTH?"

When electromagnetic radiation, like radio waves, light waves or far infrared waves travel through space they are said to make their own repeating sine wave patterns. The wavelength is simply the distance over which the wave's shape repeats. For example, red light has a shorter wavelength than near infrared, and far infrared has an even longer wavelength.

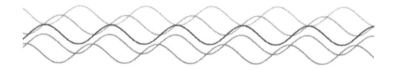

"CAN INCANDESCENT, HALOGEN OR FLUORESCENT BULBS BE USED FOR RED LIGHT THERAPY?"

Incandescent and halogen light bulbs emit as much as 35% of their total power output within the therapeutic range for light therapy.

In addition to using my red light therapy LED device daily, I've incorporated infrared heat lamps in my home as a way to enrich my environment. Proper lighting is essential for human health, and the health of all creatures. My cat, who falls asleep under them regularly, would agree.

Fluorescent bulbs are a different story. They emit some ultraviolet light but almost no red or near-infrared radiation, which is likely why many people experience unwanted side effects from exposure to these lights. Dr. Ray Peat has said the use of fluorescent lights in offices and workplaces is likely a large contributor to the epidemic of disease we see today.

"WHY ARE THE BENEFITS OF RED AND NEAR-INFRARED ARE BETTER THEN FAR-INFRARED? I READ THAT FAR INFRARED WAVES ARE SAFER FOR HUMANS IN TERM OF RADIATION EXPOSURE."

Red/near-infrared radiation (600nm to 1400nm) is absorbed by an enzyme within the mitochondria of cells called cytochrome c oxidase. This results in greater energy production by that cell. Adequate energy production is the hallmark of a healthy cell. If enough of your cells are producing energy efficiently, your body will be in good health.

Unlike red/near-infrared radiation, far infrared produces its benefit inside the body in a different way.

Far-infrared has a larger wavelength than red and near-infrared of about 1500nm-10,000nm (1mm). Instead of being absorbed by the cytochrome enzyme like red and near-infrared, far infrared improves the body's metabolism by temporarily increasing its overall temperature. Raising the body temperature by bathing in warm salty water can have a similar effect on metabolism. The reason for this is that lowering the body's overall temperature by just a degree or two can significantly lower enzymatic activity. Reduced enzymatic activity means reduced metabolic energy production. So to the extent that the body temperature is lower than ideal (98-98.6), the use of an infrared sauna will help restore the function of enzymes necessary for efficient metabolism to take place.

My parents used to have a far infrared sauna when I was living with them, so I got to use it for a period of time. At around that same time, I learned about near-infrared saunas from the book *Sauna Therapy*, and used the instructions inside the book to build myself one using PVC pipes and painters cloth. I had been aware of and concerned with the dangers of electromagnetic fields and tested emissions from both saunas using a tri-field meter. As it turns out, the EMF emissions coming from the far infrared sauna heating element were very high and coming from the near-infrared heat lamps were zero at a few inches distance.

RED LIGHT THERAPY: MIRACLE MEDICINE

"WHY DO I FEEL TINGLING DURING LIGHT THERAPY?"

According to Dr. Michael Hamblin, the 'tingling' feeling some people feel on their skin during red light therapy administration is literally the photodissociation of nitric oxide from the cytochrome c oxidase enzyme taking place inside cells.

"I WANT TO USE THE LIGHT FOR WRINKLES ON MY FACE AND ARTHRITIS ON MY ANKLES, BUT WANT TO AVOID GROWING HAIR ON THOSE PARTS OF MY BODY. I HAVE HAIR ON MY FACE THAT I DO NOT WANT TO GROW AND HAD LASER HAIR REMOVAL ON MY LEGS, BUT I HAVE ARTHRITIS THERE. WILL THE RED LIGHT CAUSE HAIR TO GROW IN THOSE PLACES?"

The way laser hair removal works is by damaging the hair follicles repeatedly until they can no longer produce hair. Red light will assist your body in repairing the damaged follicles caused by the laser hair removal. Based on this, applying red light to your face and legs will likely reduce wrinkles, pain and inflammation, but unfortunately, will likely also improve the rate of hair growth in both of those places.

RED LIGHT THERAPY: MIRACLE MEDICINE

"IS RED LIGHT EFFECTIVE FOR ROSACEA?"

Since red light improves metabolism, or a cell's ability to produce energy, and since adequate energy production can be considered the hallmark of cellular health, there are likely no cells or tissues that will not benefit from red light.

A review on red light for skin conditions reports "Several studies reported effectiveness and safety of LED therapy in photo-aged skin [22–26]. LED therapy efficacy was also reported for instance in wound-healing [28, 29] as in psoriasis [30–32] and rosacea [33–36]."

"IS *PULSED* RED LIGHT THERAPY EFFECTIVE?"

Instead of simply repeating someone else's findings to you, I decided to read everything I could find on pulsed red light therapy so I could give you a proper answer. Below I share with you my findings.

Pulsed red light therapy is basically a 'flickering' on-and-off of red light at specific pulse frequencies. Pulsed red light therapy affects cells in the same way as traditional 'continuous wave' red light therapy[1-2] - by enhancing cellular ATP production within the mitochondria of cells.

When comparing the value of pulsed wave vs. continuous wave red light therapy, there is conflicting evidence. Some studies indicate that pulsed wave is more effective, and others indicate that continuous wave is more effective.

For example, a 2004 study by Saudi Arabian scientists compared the effects of continuous wave red light therapy with pulsed red light therapy on burn wounds in rats. The pulse frequencies they tested were 100Hz, 200Hz, 300Hz, 400Hz and 500Hz, and the study found that continuous wave was more effective than 100Hz pulsed wave.[3]

	Pulse Frequency	Healing
Pulsed Wave	100 Hz 200 Hz 300 Hz 400 Hz 500 Hz	4.32 % 3.21 % 3.83 % 2.22 % 1.73 %
Continuous Wave	-	4.81 %

Note: Pulse frequency is measured in a unit called Hertz, which is the number of 'on-off' cycles per second.

Dr. Michael Hamblin from Harvard University has written an extensive review on pulsed red and near-infrared light therapy in which they analyzed the effects of a wide range of frequencies including everything from:

- 2-3 Hertz

- Tens of Hertz

- Hundreds of Hertz

- Thousands of Hertz (Kilohertz)

- Tens of thousands of Hertz (Tens of Kilohertz)

- Hundreds of thousands of Hertz (Hundreds of Kilohertz)

- Megahertz (Thousands of Kilohertz/Millions of Hertz)

What did Hamblin and his group conclude from their research? "The conclusion was if you're going to do pulsing, don't make the frequency too high because cells just get confused," said Hamblin in an interview.[4] If you're going to do pulsing, continued Hamblin, anywhere between 10Hz and 100Hz might be useful.

There are a couple unique properties about pulsed red light which I think are worth mentioning. One is that pulsed red light can penetrate through skin and skin barriers, such as pigment, more easily than continuous wave red light.[5-6] Red and particularly near-infrared light are already effective at accessing cells deep inside the body but *pulsed* red and near-infrared light may be even better at reaching deep target tissues.

Another unique property of pulsed red light is that it transfers less heat to tissues, since the light is 'off' as much as it is 'on'. This can be useful for heat sensitive tissues, such as the brain or testicles, whose function are reduced by exposure to excessive heat.[7-8]

PULSED RED LIGHT THERAPY CONCLUSION

Continuous wave red light therapy is already remarkably effective, and some evidence suggests that pulsing it may make it slightly more effective. Pulsed red light has the unique ability to reach tissues deeper into the body and cause less tissue heating, which can be advantageous for certain disorders. However, given the fact that pulsed red light therapy devices are more expensive to manufacture and are more susceptible to malfunction and reduced longevity from the constant on and off cycles, continuous wave red light therapy seems to be the most practical and efficient.

"I WAS WONDERING ABOUT THE TESTIMONIAL FROM KAYA WHO HAD GREAT SUCCESS WITH HER VISION – DO YOU HAVE ANY IDEA OF THE PROTOCOL SHE USED TO IMPROVE HER EYESIGHT?"

While I don't have the exact protocol Kaya used to successfully improve her vision with red light therapy, I can give you a protocol that will give you the absolute best chance of success.

The best way to improve vision using red light is to apply it directly to your eyes directly and also to your fully body. All health issues are holistic in nature and full-body light therapy can help shift the metabolism of the entire body in a positive direction. I recommend 15 minutes per day directly in the eyes (morning) and 15 minutes full body session (before bed) using the following positioning:

- Lay on your side in the fetal position, on your bed or on a towel on the floor, fully unclothed
- Place the light 1-2 feet away aimed at your abdomen. (The light should reach all skin exposed from your upper legs to your stomach and chest, as well as your upper arms.)
- Set a timer for about 15-20 minutes then relax and enjoy

After following this protocol for a couple weeks, visit your optometrist for an eye exam. You will likely see results for not only your vision but also for your overall health (i.e. improved energy, vitality, brain function, etc).

I hope you enjoyed this chapter and that it has answered some of your own questions about red and near-infrared light therapy.

CONCLUSION

REDEFINING MEDICINE

WHILE TRADITIONAL MEDICINE HAS FOREVER involved the administration of plant and animal foods derived from nature, a western medical establishment was born in the mid-20th century which redefined the term 'medicine.' Suddenly the use of toxic man-made drugs and dangerous surgical procedures became the predominant forms of therapy. This change was essential for the establishment of a system of healthcare based on profit, since substances found in nature cannot be patented.

Within this for-profit healthcare system, the more toxic and dangerous drugs or treatments are, the better they are as products. This is because highly toxic drugs result in any number of side effects, which render patients in need of more drugs to treat those side effects. Modern medicine's profit-before-patient ethos has resulted in millions of unnecessary deaths, incalculable suffering and has generated the greatest public health disaster in history. Thankfully, the world is becoming increasingly aware of the fact that a medical system which seeks profit has no interest in healing people.

When Dr. Gary Null and his team of scientists reviewed all existing research on doctor-induced injury and death in 2002, they didn't know exactly what they would find. Their goal was simply to discover the truth about whether or not the medical system was ultimately harming us or healing us. The publication of their study *Death by Medicine* marked a monumental turning point in medicine. It was the moment when a tragic yet necessary truth was realized: Modern medicine is causing *much* more harm than good. Is anyone surprised to hear that these findings were not broadcast publically by the drug company-funded mainstream media?

Of the thousands of drugs and surgical procedures offered by the medical establishment today, none address the root cause of disease. Instead of focusing on the origins of the problem, they provide only temporary relief of a patient's symptoms. This business model is fantastic for generating enormous profits, but as previously mentioned, as long as the primary directive of the medical industry is revenue, the 'medicines' it offers will never truly provide healing. This type of medical system has rendered populations of people never quite healthy and repeatedly coming back for more drugs and surgeries.

What do you do when you find yourself living in a world in which the medical system that exists to serve you is broken? A world where there's almost nothing a doctor can do for you that won't make your health worse? A world where mainstream medicine kills more people than it helps? Simple. You change it.

PARADIGM SHIFT: FROM DRUGS AND SURGERIES TO FOOD AND LIGHT

Visit a medical doctor and you risk being diagnosed with one or more of the 30,000+ 'officially' classified diseases. Healthcare professionals and the public have been conditioned over many decades that tens of thousands of diseases exist. For pharmaceutical manufacturers, the invention of every new disease means additional revenue from at least one new product. The more diseases that are claimed to exist, the more profit can be made. As Buckminster Fuller once wrote, 'the truth is always beautiful and simple' - and the truth is that only one disease exists: A malfunctioning cell.

The primary reason why drug and surgical based therapies have been such a colossal failure is, of course, that it's not for lack of poison or knives that cells begin to malfunction. Modern science has established that the genesis of disease in the body is almost universally the result of a disruption in cellular metabolism. A cell that's unable to metabolize food into energy efficiently might be the most accurate definition of an unhealthy cell. When a large number of cells in the body aren't generating sufficient energy, in the form of adenosine triphosphate (ATP), then the organism as a whole is unhealthy. This decline in energy production is the prime cause of the symptoms experienced by the patient. These symptoms are typically what compel people to visit their doctors, who then diagnose patients with a specific disease and prescribe specific drugs or surgeries. Although the symptomatic relief afforded by some drugs and surgeries are of benefit to patients in the short term, in the long term the root cause of the problem is only made worse by these interventions.

Conversely, when you avoid the things that poison cellular metabolic processes (environmental toxins & injury), and expose the body to factors essential for efficient metabolism (nutrients and light), malfunctioning cells begin to function correctly, symptoms disappear and total body health is restored.

THE RED LIGHT REVOLUTION

Over 50,000 scientific studies to date have shown that red and near-infrared light can effectively restore and enhance the function of virtually any cell or tissues in the body. According to the research, red light therapy can help with literally dozens of diseases and conditions. But since red light is an antioxidant and a non-tissue-specific healing accelerant, the reality is there are probably no ailments that cannot benefit from it. What's more, not a single negative side effect to date has been reported in the scientific literature.

It is now understood that enzymes within cells absorb light in the red and near-infrared ends of the spectrum – and when they do, cellular metabolism is enhanced. This enhancement in energy production allows the body to accomplish all the vital functions it needs not only for survival, but for peak functioning and performance. Health has always been *a matter of energy*.

No medicine in the world has the track record of red light therapy for safety and efficacy. If it weren't for the fact that red light devices are inexpensive and can last for decades, the pharmaceutical industry would probably be hailing red light therapy the greatest therapy ever discovered. If you could pack photons of red light into a pill, it would undoubtedly be a billion-dollar blockbuster drug. But doctors will probably never tell you that unless they have an expensive red light therapy machine that you can pay them to use regularly - which is why I have written this book. LED technology has made red light therapy inexpensive and available to virtually everybody from the comfort of their own home.

The solariums that ancient Egyptians used for healing have not only survived the rigors of modern science, but they have been vindicated by it. The precise physiological mechanisms of red light on the organism have been discovered and presented in this book in complete detail.

The final frontier in red light research has been achieved, and no more science is needed for humanity to begin reaping the benefits of red light therapy, today. Once the red light revolution finishes sweeping the earth, all toxic and ineffective medicines in its path will be replaced, and red light will be hailed as one of the safest and most miraculous medicines ever discovered.

REFERENCES

WHY YOU SHOULD READ THIS BOOK

1. BioOptics World. 2013. FDA approves LED light therapy device from BioPhotas. Available: https://www.bioopticsworld.com/articles/2013/01/fda-approves-led-light-therapy-device-from-biophotas.html [February 10th, 2018].

2. Medical Daily. 2014. FDA Approves iGrow, A Low-Leven Laser Therapy Device That Stimulates Hair Growth In Med. Available: http://www.medicaldaily.com/fda-approves-igrow-low-level-laser-therapy-device-stimulates-hair-growth-men-304890 [February 10th, 2018].

3. BMJ Group Blogs. 2016. Too Much Medicine-Prescription drugs are the third leading cause of death. Available: http://blogs.bmj.com/ce/2016/06/16/too-much-medicine-prescription-drugs-are-the-third-leading-cause-of-death/ [February 10th, 2018].

4. Starfield B. Is US health really the best in the world? JAMA. 2000;284(4):483-485.

5. Null G, Dean C, Feldman M, Rasio D, Smith D. Death By Medicine. 2003. Available: http://www.webdc.com/pdfs/deathbymedicine.pdf [February 10, 2018].

History

1. NobelPrize.org. Neils Ryberg Finsen – Biographical. Available: https://www.nobelprize.org/nobel_prizes/medicine/laureates/1903/finsen-bio.html [February 10th, 2018].

2. Hamblin MR. Shining light on the head: Photobiomodulation for brain disorders. BBA Clin. 2016;6:113-124.

3. Mester E, Szende B, Gärtner P. [The effect of laser beams on the growth of hair in mice]. Radiobiol Radiother (Berl). 1968;9(5):621-6.

4. Chung H, Dai T, Sharma SK, Huang YY, Carroll JD, Hamblin MR. The nuts and bolts of low-level laser (light) therapy. Ann Biomed Eng. 2012;40(2):516-33.

5. New Scientist. 1987. The 'healing laser' comes into the limelight. Available: https://books.google.ca/books?id=qxwPsfm2RS8 C&pg=PA32&redir_esc=y#v=onepage&q&f=fals e [February 10th, 2018].

RED AND NEAR-INFRARED RADIATION

1. Schnatz PF, Manson JE. Vitamin D and cardiovascular disease: an appraisal of the evidence. Clin Chem. 2014;60(4):600-9.

2. Valtsu's Blog. 2017. The Therapeutic Effects of Red and Near-Infrared Light (2017). Available: https://valtsus.blogspot.ca/2017/05/the-therapeutic-effects-of-red-and-near.html [February 10th, 2018].

3. Hong Kong Far Infrared Rays Association. Fundamentals of Far-Infrared. Available: http://www.hkfira.org/webhp/upload/fir_105/2 0090828-02%20-%20Prof%20Cheah%20-%20HKBU%20-%20Fundamental%20of%20FIR.pdf [February 10th, 2018].

THE SCIENCE OF LIGHT THERAPY

1. De brito A, Alves AN, Ribeiro BG, et al. Effect of photobiomodulation on connective tissue remodeling and regeneration of skeletal muscle in elderly rats. Lasers Med Sci. 2017.

2. Trawitzki BF, Lilge L, De figueiredo FAT, Macedo AP, Issa JPM. Low-intensity laser therapy efficacy

evaluation in mice subjected to acute arthritis condition. J Photochem Photobiol B, Biol. 2017;174:126-132.

3. Meyer DM, Chen Y, Zivin JA. Dose-finding study of phototherapy on stroke outcome in a rabbit model of ischemic stroke. Neurosci Lett. 2016;630:254-8.

4. Figurová M, Ledecký V, Karasová M, et al. Histological Assessment of a Combined Low-Level Laser/Light-Emitting Diode Therapy (685 nm/470 nm) for Sutured Skin Incisions in a Porcine Model: A Short Report. Photomed Laser Surg. 2016;34(2):53-5.

5. Oron U, Yaakobi T, Oron A, et al. Low-energy laser irradiation reduces formation of scar tissue after myocardial infarction in rats and dogs. Circulation. 2001;103(2):296-301.

6. Darlot F, Moro C, El massri N, et al. Near-infrared light is neuroprotective in a monkey model of Parkinson disease. Ann Neurol. 2016;79(1):59-75.

7. Blatt A, Elbaz-greener GA, Tuby H, et al. Low-Level Laser Therapy to the Bone Marrow Reduces Scarring and Improves Heart Function Post-Acute Myocardial Infarction in the Pig. Photomed Laser Surg. 2016;34(11):516-524.

8. Freddo AL, Hübler R, De castro-beck CA, Heitz C, De oliveira MG. A preliminary study of hardness and modulus of elasticity in sheep mandibles submitted to distraction osteogenesis

and low-level laser therapy. Med Oral Patol Oral Cir Bucal. 2012;17(1):e102-7.

9. Petersen SL, Botes C, Olivier A, Guthrie AJ. The effect of low level laser therapy (LLLT) on wound healing in horses. Equine Vet J. 1999;31(3):228-31.

10. Ghamsari SM, Taguchi K, Abe N, Acorda JA, Sato M, Yamada H. Evaluation of low level laser therapy on primary healing of experimentally induced full thickness teat wounds in dairy cattle. Vet Surg. 1997;26(2):114-20.

11. Mezawa S, Iwata K, Naito K, Kamogawa H. The possible analgesic effect of soft-laser irradiation on heat nociceptors in the cat tongue. Arch Oral Biol. 1988;33(9):693-4.

12. Byrnes KR, Barna L, Chenault VM, et al. Photobiomodulation improves cutaneous wound healing in an animal model of type II diabetes. Photomed Laser Surg. 2004;22(4):281-90.

13. Iyomasa DM, Garavelo I, Iyomasa MM, Watanabe IS, Issa JP. Ultrastructural analysis of the low level laser therapy effects on the lesioned anterior tibial muscle in the gerbil. Micron. 2009;40(4):413-8.

14. Maleki Sh, Kamrava SK, Sharifi D, et al. Effect of local irradiation with 630 and 860 nm low-level lasers on tympanic membrane perforation repair in guinea pigs. J Laryngol Otol. 2013;127(3):260-4.

15. Comelekoglu U, Bagis S, Buyukakilli B, Sahin G, Erdogan C. Electrophysiologic effect of gallium arsenide laser on frog gastrocnemius muscle. Lasers Surg Med. 2002;30(3):221-6.

16. Powner MB, Salt TE, Hogg C, Jeffery G. Improving Mitochondrial Function Protects Bumblebees from Neonicotinoid Pesticides. PLoS ONE. 2016;11(11):e0166531.

17. Begum R, Calaza K, Kam JH, Salt TE, Hogg C, Jeffery G. Near-infrared light increases ATP, extends lifespan and improves mobility in aged Drosophila melanogaster. Biol Lett. 2015;11(3).

18. Amaroli A, Gambardella C, Ferrando S, et al. The Effect of Photobiomodulation on the Sea Urchin Paracentrotus lividus (Echinodermata) Using Higher-Fluence on Fertilization, Embryogenesis, and Larval Development: An In Vitro Study. Photomed Laser Surg. 2017;35(3):127-135.

19. Contzen Pereira. Improved cognitive functions and behavioural response after exposure to low-level near-infrared laser in snails (Ariophanta laevipes). 2017; 5(1): 169-176.

20. Duggett, NA. Photobiomodulation in Animal Models of Ageing and Alzheimer's Disease. *Durham University*. 2013.

21. Amaroli A, Ferrando S, Hanna R, et al. The photobiomodulation effect of higher-fluence 808-nm laser therapy with a flat-top handpiece on the wound healing of the earthworm Dendrobaena veneta: a brief report. Lasers Med Sci. 2018;33(1):221-225.

22. Wu HP, Persinger MA. Increased mobility and stem-cell proliferation rate in Dugesia tigrina induced by 880nm light emitting diode. J Photochem Photobiol B, Biol. 2011;102(2):156-60.

23. Bjordal JM, Lopes-martins RA, Iversen VV. A randomised, placebo controlled trial of low level laser therapy for activated Achilles tendinitis with microdialysis measurement of peritendinous prostaglandin E2 concentrations. Br J Sports Med. 2006;40(1):76-80.

24. Marcos RL, Arnold G, Magnenet V, Rahouadj R, Magdalou J, Lopes-martins RÁ. Biomechanical and biochemical protective effect of low-level laser therapy for Achilles tendinitis. J Mech Behav Biomed Mater. 2014;29:272-85.

25. Tumilty S, Munn J, Abbott JH, Mcdonough S, Hurley DA, Baxter GD. Laser therapy in the treatment of achilles tendinopathy: a pilot study. Photomed Laser Surg. 2008;26(1):25-30.

26. Stergioulas A, Stergioula M, Aarskog R, Lopes-martins RA, Bjordal JM. Effects of low-level laser therapy and eccentric exercises in the treatment of recreational athletes with chronic achilles tendinopathy. Am J Sports Med. 2008;36(5):881-7.

27. Charakida A, Seaton ED, Charakida M, Mouser P, Avgerinos A, Chu AC. Phototherapy in the treatment of acne vulgaris: what is its role?. Am J Clin Dermatol. 2004;5(4):211-6.

28. Na JI, Suh DH. Red light phototherapy alone is effective for acne vulgaris: randomized, single-blinded clinical trial. Dermatol Surg. 2007;33(10):1228-33.

29. Aziz-jalali MH, Tabaie SM, Djavid GE. Comparison of Red and Infrared Low-level Laser

REFERENCES

Therapy in the Treatment of Acne Vulgaris. Indian J Dermatol. 2012;57(2):128-30.

30. Kerr CM, Lowe PB, Spielholz NI. Low level laser for the stimulation of acupoints for smoking cessation: a double blind, placebo controlled randomized trial and semi structured interviews. J Chin Med. 2008;86:46-51.

31. Ivandic BT, Ivandic T. Low-level laser therapy improves visual acuity in adolescent and adult patients with amblyopia. Photomed Laser Surg. 2012;30(3):167-71.

32. Olk RJ, Friberg TR, Stickney KL, et al. Therapeutic benefits of infrared (810-nm) diode laser macular grid photocoagulation in prophylactic treatment of nonexudative age-related macular degeneration: two-year results of a randomized pilot study. Ophthalmology. 1999;106(11):2082-90.

33. Ivandic BT, Ivandic T. Low-level laser therapy improves vision in patients with age-related macular degeneration. Photomed Laser Surg. 2008;26(3):241-5.

34. Saltmarche AE, Naeser MA, Ho KF, Hamblin MR, Lim L. Significant Improvement in Cognition in Mild to Moderately Severe Dementia Cases Treated with Transcranial Plus Intranasal Photobiomodulation: Case Series Report. Photomed Laser Surg. 2017;35(8):432-441.

35. Aggarwal H, Singh MP, Nahar P, Mathur H, Gv S. Efficacy of low-level laser therapy in treatment of recurrent aphthous ulcers - a sham controlled, split

mouth follow up study. J Clin Diagn Res. 2014;8(2):218-21.

36. Vale FA, Moreira MS, De almeida FC, Ramalho KM. Low-level laser therapy in the treatment of recurrent aphthous ulcers: a systematic review. ScientificWorldJournal. 2015;2015:150412.

37. Suter VGA, Sjölund S, Bornstein MM. Effect of laser on pain relief and wound healing of recurrent aphthous stomatitis: a systematic review. Lasers Med Sci. 2017;32(4):953-963.

38. Alayat MS, Elsodany AM, El fiky AA. Efficacy of high and low level laser therapy in the treatment of Bell's palsy: a randomized double blind placebo-controlled trial. Lasers Med Sci. 2014;29(1):335-42.

39. Fontana CR, Bagnato VS. Low-level laser therapy in pediatric Bell's palsy: case report in a three-year-old child. J Altern Complement Med. 2013;19(4):376-82.

40. Ordahan B, Karahan AY. Role of low-level laser therapy added to facial expression exercises in patients with idiopathic facial (Bell's) palsy. Lasers Med Sci. 2017;32(4):931-936.

41. Chang WD, Wu JH, Wang HJ, Jiang JA. Therapeutic outcomes of low-level laser therapy for closed bone fracture in the human wrist and hand. Photomed Laser Surg. 2014;32(4):212-8.

42. Quirk BJ, Sannagowdara K, Buchmann EV, Jensen ES, Gregg DC, Whelan HT. Effect of near-infrared light oncellular ATP production of osteoblasts and fibroblasts and on fracture healing

with intramedullary fixation. J Clin Orthop Trauma. 2016;7(4):234-241.

43. Liu X, Lyon R, Meier HT, Thometz J, Haworth ST. Effect of lower-level laser therapy on rabbit tibial fracture. Photomed Laser Surg. 2007;25(6):487-94.

44. Gaida K, Koller R, Isler C, et al. Low Level Laser Therapy--a conservative approach to the burn scar?. Burns. 2004;30(4):362-7.

45. Al-maweri SA, Javed F, Kalakonda B, Alaizari NA, Al-soneidar W, Al-akwa A. Efficacy of low level laser therapy in the treatment of burning mouth syndrome: A systematic review. Photodiagnosis Photodyn Ther. 2017;17:188-193.

46. Valenzuela S, Lopez-jornet P. Effects of low-level laser therapy on burning mouth syndrome. J Oral Rehabil. 2017;44(2):125-132.

47. Chang WD, Wu JH, Jiang JA, Yeh CY, Tsai CT. Carpal tunnel syndrome treated with a diode laser: a controlled treatment of the transverse carpal ligament. Photomed Laser Surg. 2008;26(6):551-7.

48. Li ZJ, Wang Y, Zhang HF, Ma XL, Tian P, Huang Y. Effectiveness of low-level laser on carpal tunnel syndrome: A meta-analysis of previously reported randomized trials. Medicine (Baltimore). 2016;95(31):e4424.

49. Avci P, Nyame TT, Gupta GK, Sadasivam M, Hamblin MR. Low-level laser therapy for fat layer reduction: a comprehensive review. Lasers Surg Med. 2013;45(6):349-57.

50. Bjordal JM, Couppé C, Chow RT, Tunér J, Ljunggren EA. A systematic review of low level laser therapy with location-specific doses for pain from chronic joint disorders. Aust J Physiother. 2003;49(2):107-16.

51. Vargas E, Barrett DW, Saucedo CL, et al. Beneficial neurocognitive effects of transcranial laser in older adults. Lasers Med Sci. 2017;32(5):1153-1162.

52. Barrett DW, Gonzalez-lima F. Transcranial infrared laser stimulation produces beneficial cognitive and emotional effects in humans. Neuroscience. 2013;230:13-23.

53. Hwang J, Castelli DM, Gonzalez-lima F. Cognitive enhancement by transcranial laser stimulation and acute aerobic exercise. Lasers Med Sci. 2016;31(6):1151-60.

54. Gonzalez-lima F, Barrett DW. Augmentation of cognitive brain functions with transcranial lasers. Front Syst Neurosci. 2014;8:36.

55. De paula eduardo C, Aranha AC, Simões A, et al. Laser treatment of recurrent herpes labialis: a literature review. Lasers Med Sci. 2014;29(4):1517-29.

56. Muñoz sanchez PJ, Capote femenías JL, Díaz tejeda A, Tunér J. The effect of 670-nm low laser therapy on herpes simplex type 1. Photomed Laser Surg. 2012;30(1):37-40.

57. Miranda EF, De oliveira LV, Antonialli FC, Vanin AA, De carvalho Pde T, Leal-junior EC. Phototherapy with combination of super-pulsed

laser and light-emitting diodes is beneficial in improvement of muscular performance (strength and muscular endurance), dyspnea, and fatigue sensation in patients with chronic obstructive pulmonary disease. Lasers Med Sci. 2015;30(1):437-43.

58. Gokmenoglu C, Ozmeric N, Erguder I, Elgun S. The effect of light-emitting diode photobiomodulation on implant stability and biochemical markers in peri-implant crevicular fluid. Photomed Laser Surg. 2014;32(3):138-45.

59. Ko Y, Park J, Kim C, Park J, Baek SH, Kook YA. Treatment of dentin hypersensitivity with a low-level laser-emitting toothbrush: double-blind randomised clinical trial of efficacy and safety. J Oral Rehabil. 2014;41(7):523-31.

60. Schiffer F, Johnston AL, Ravichandran C, Polcari A, Teicher MH, Webb RH, Hamblin MR. Psychological benefits 2 and 4 weeks after a single treatment with near infrared light to the forehead: a pilot study of 10 patients with major depression and anxiety. Behav Brain Functions. 2009; 5:46.

61. Henderson TA, Morries LD. Multi-Watt Near-Infrared Phototherapy for the Treatment of Comorbid Depression: An Open-Label Single-Arm Study. Front Psychiatry. 2017;8:187.

62. Barrett DW, Gonzalez-lima F. Transcranial infrared laser stimulation produces beneficial cognitive and emotional effects in humans. Neuroscience. 2013;230:13-23.

63. Tchanque-fossuo CN, Ho D, Dahle SE, Koo E, Isseroff RR, Jagdeo J. Low-level Light Therapy for Treatment of Diabetic Foot Ulcer: A Review of Clinical Experiences. J Drugs Dermatol. 2016;15(7):843-8.

64. Tchanque-fossuo CN, Ho D, Dahle SE, et al. A systematic review of low-level light therapy for treatment of diabetic foot ulcer. Wound Repair Regen. 2016;24(2):418-26.

65. Lončar B, Stipetić MM, Baričević M, Risović D. The effect of low-level laser therapy on salivary glands in patients with xerostomia. Photomed Laser Surg. 2011;29(3):171-5.

66. Pavlić V. [The effects of low-level laser therapy on xerostomia (mouth dryness)]. Med Pregl. 2012;65(5-6):247-50.

67. Vidović juras D, Lukac J, Cekić-arambasin A, et al. Effects of low-level laser treatment on mouth dryness. Coll Antropol. 2010;34(3):1039-43.

68. Shin YI, Kim NG, Park KJ, Kim DW, Hong GY, Shin BC. Skin adhesive low-level light therapy for dysmenorrhoea: a randomized, double-blind, placebo-controlled, pilot trial. Arch Gynecol Obstet. 2012;286(4):947-52.

69. Hong GY, Shin BC, Park SN, et al. Randomized controlled trial of the efficacy and safety of self-adhesive low-level light therapy in women with primary dysmenorrhea. Int J Gynaecol Obstet. 2016;133(1):37-42.

70. Bjordal JM, Lopes-martins RA, Joensen J, et al. A systematic review with procedural assessments and

meta-analysis of low level laser therapy in lateral elbow tendinopathy (tennis elbow). BMC Musculoskelet Disord. 2008;9:75.

71. Antonialli FC, De marchi T, Tomazoni SS, et al. Phototherapy in skeletal muscle performance and recovery after exercise: effect of combination of super-pulsed laser and light-emitting diodes. Lasers Med Sci. 2014;29(6):1967-76.

72. Miranda EF, Vanin AA, Tomazoni SS, et al. Using Pre-Exercise Photobiomodulation Therapy Combining Super-Pulsed Lasers and Light-Emitting Diodes to Improve Performance in Progressive Cardiopulmonary Exercise Tests. J Athl Train. 2016;51(2):129-35.

73. Leal-junior EC, Vanin AA, Miranda EF, De carvalho Pde T, Dal corso S, Bjordal JM. Effect of phototherapy (low-level laser therapy and light-emitting diode therapy) on exercise performance and markers of exercise recovery: a systematic review with meta-analysis. Lasers Med Sci. 2015;30(2):925-39.

74. Ferraresi C, Beltrame T, Fabrizzi F, et al. Muscular pre-conditioning using light-emitting diode therapy (LEDT) for high-intensity exercise: a randomized double-blind placebo-controlled trial with a single elite runner. Physiother Theory Pract. 2015;31(5):354-61.

75. Aver vanin A, De marchi T, Tomazoni SS, et al. Pre-Exercise Infrared Low-Level Laser Therapy (810 nm) in Skeletal Muscle Performance and Postexercise Recovery in Humans, What Is the

Optimal Dose? A Randomized, Double-Blind, Placebo-Controlled Clinical Trial. Photomed Laser Surg. 2016;34(10):473-482.

76. De souza RC, De sousa ET, Scudine KG, et al. Low-level laser therapy and anesthetic infiltration for orofacial pain in patients with fibromyalgia: a randomized clinical trial. Med Oral Patol Oral Cir Bucal. 2018;23(1):e65-e71.

77. Ruaro JA, Fréz AR, Ruaro MB, Nicolau RA. Low-level laser therapy to treat fibromyalgia. Lasers Med Sci. 2014;29(6):1815-9.

78. Page MJ, Green S, Kramer S, Johnston RV, Mcbain B, Buchbinder R. Electrotherapy modalities for adhesive capsulitis (frozen shoulder). Cochrane Database Syst Rev. 2014;(10):CD011324.

79. Ivandic BT, Ivandic T. Effects of Photobiomodulation Therapy on Patients with Primary Open Angle Glaucoma: A Pilot Study. Photomed Laser Surg. 2015;

80. Avci P, Gupta GK, Clark J, Wikonkal N, Hamblin MR. Low-level laser (light) therapy (LLLT) for treatment of hair loss. Lasers Surg Med. 2014;46(2):144-51.

81. Zarei M, Wikramanayake TC, Falto-aizpurua L, Schachner LA, Jimenez JJ. Low level laser therapy and hair regrowth: an evidence-based review. Lasers Med Sci. 2016;31(2):363-71.

82. Toida M, Watanabe F, Goto K, Shibata T. Usefulness of low-level laser for control of painful

stomatitis in patients with hand-foot-and-mouth disease. J Clin Laser Med Surg. 2003;21(6):363-7.

83. Höfling DB, Chavantes MC, Juliano AG, et al. Low-level laser in the treatment of patients with hypothyroidism induced by chronic autoimmune thyroiditis: a randomized, placebo-controlled clinical trial. Lasers Med Sci. 2013;28(3):743-53.

84. Chung H, Dai T, Sharma SK, Huang YY, Carroll JD, Hamblin MR. The nuts and bolts of low-level laser (light) therapy. Ann Biomed Eng. 2012;40(2):516-33.

85. Höfling DB, Chavantes MC, Juliano AG, et al. Low-level laser therapy in chronic autoimmune thyroiditis: a pilot study. Lasers Surg Med. 2010;42(6):589-96.

86. Al-maweri SA, Kalakonda B, Al-soneidar WA, Al-shamiri HM, Alakhali MS, Alaizari N. Efficacy of low-level laser therapy in management of symptomatic oral lichen planus: a systematic review. Lasers Med Sci. 2017;32(6):1429-1437.

87. Huang Z, Ma J, Chen J, Shen B, Pei F, Kraus VB. The effectiveness of low-level laser therapy for nonspecific chronic low back pain: a systematic review and meta-analysis. Arthritis Res Ther. 2015;17:360.

88. Glazov G, Yelland M, Emery J. Low-level laser therapy for chronic non-specific low back pain: a meta-analysis of randomised controlled trials. Acupunct Med. 2016;34(5):328-341.

89. Yousefi-nooraie R, Schonstein E, Heidari K, et al. Low level laser therapy for nonspecific low-back

pain. Cochrane Database Syst Rev. 2007;(2):CD005107.

90. Omar MT, Shaheen AA, Zafar H. A systematic review of the effect of low-level laser therapy in the management of breast cancer-related lymphedema. Support Care Cancer. 2012;20(11):2977-84.

91. E lima MT, E lima JG, De andrade MF, Bergmann A. Low-level laser therapy in secondary lymphedema after breast cancer: systematic review. Lasers Med Sci. 2014;29(3):1289-95.

92. Smoot B, Chiavola-larson L, Lee J, Manibusan H, Allen DD. Effect of low-level laser therapy on pain and swelling in women with breast cancer-related lymphedema: a systematic review and meta-analysis. J Cancer Surviv. 2015;9(2):287-304.

93. Mortazavi H, Khalighi H, Goljanian A, Noormohammadi R, Mojahedi S, Sabour S. Intra-oral low level laser therapy in chronic maxillary sinusitis: A new and effective recommended technique. J Clin Exp Dent. 2015;7(5):e557-62.

94. Ferraresi C, Huang YY, Hamblin MR. Photobiomodulation in human muscle tissue: an advantage in sports performance?. J Biophotonics. 2016;9(11-12):1273-1299.

95. Baroni BM, Rodrigues R, Freire BB, Franke Rde A, Geremia JM, Vaz MA. Effect of low-level laser therapy on muscle adaptation to knee extensor eccentric training. Eur J Appl Physiol. 2015;115(3):639-47.

REFERENCES

96. Ferraresi C, Huang YY, Hamblin MR. Photobiomodulation in human muscle tissue: an advantage in sports performance?. J Biophotonics. 2016;9(11-12):1273-1299.

97. Law D, Mcdonough S, Bleakley C, Baxter GD, Tumilty S. Laser acupuncture for treating musculoskeletal pain: a systematic review with meta-analysis. J Acupunct Meridian Stud. 2015;8(1):2-16.

98. Chow RT, Johnson MI, Lopes-Martins RAB, Bjordal JM. Efficacy of low-level laser therapy in the management of neck pain: a systematic review and meta-analysis of randomized placebo or active-treatment controlled trials. The Lancet. 2009; 374(9705):1897-1908.

99. Kadhim-saleh A, Maganti H, Ghert M, Singh S, Farrokhyar F. Is low-level laser therapy in relieving neck pain effective? Systematic review and meta-analysis. Rheumatol Int. 2013;33(10):2493-501.

100. Ebid AA, El-kafy EM, Alayat MS. Effect of pulsed Nd:YAG laser in the treatment of neuropathic foot ulcers in children with spina bifida: a randomized controlled study. Photomed Laser Surg. 2013;31(12):565-70.

101. Coca KP, Marcacine KO, Gamba MA, Corrêa L, Aranha AC, Abrão AC. Efficacy of Low-Level Laser Therapy in Relieving Nipple Pain in Breastfeeding Women: A Triple-Blind, Randomized, Controlled Trial. Pain Manag Nurs. 2016;17(4):281-9.

102.   Chaves ME, Araújo AR, Santos SF, Pinotti M, Oliveira LS. LED phototherapy improves healing of nipple trauma: a pilot study. Photomed Laser Surg. 2012;30(3):172-8.

103.   Sene-fiorese M, Duarte FO, De aquino junior AE, et al. The potential of phototherapy to reduce body fat, insulin resistance and "metabolic inflexibility" related to obesity in women undergoing weight loss treatment. Lasers Surg Med. 2015;47(8):634-42.

104.   Duarte FO, Sene-Fiorese M, Eduardo de Aquino Junior A, Campos RMS, Masquio DCL, Tock L, Duarte ACGO, Damaso AR, Bagnato VS, Parizotto NA. Can low-level laser therapy (LLLT) associated with an aerobic plus resistance training change the cardiometabolic risk in obese women? A placebo-controlled clinical trial. J Photochem Photobiol. 2015; 153: 103-110.

105.   Mcrae E, Boris J. Independent evaluation of low-level laser therapy at 635 nm for non-invasive body contouring of the waist, hips, and thighs. Lasers Surg Med. 2013;45(1):1-7.

106.   Eduardo Fde P, Bezinelli LM, De carvalho DL, et al. Oral mucositis in pediatric patients undergoing hematopoietic stem cell transplantation: clinical outcomes in a context of specialized oral care using low-level laser therapy. Pediatr Transplant. 2015;19(3):316-25.

107.   Spivakovsky S. Low level laser therapy may reduce risk of oral mucositis. Evid Based Dent. 2015;16(2):49.

108.   He M, Zhang B, Shen N, Wu N, Sun J. A systematic review and meta-analysis of the effect of low-level laser therapy (LLLT) on chemotherapy-induced oral mucositis in pediatric and young patients. Eur J Pediatr. 2018;177(1):7-17.

109.   Ren C, Mcgrath C, Yang Y. The effectiveness of low-level diode laser therapy on orthodontic pain management: a systematic review and meta-analysis. Lasers Med Sci. 2015;30(7):1881-93.

110.   Li FJ, Zhang JY, Zeng XT, Guo Y. Low-level laser therapy for orthodontic pain: a systematic review. Lasers Med Sci. 2015;30(6):1789-803.

111.   Fleming PS, Strydom H, Katsaros C, et al. Non-pharmacological interventions for alleviating pain during orthodontic treatment. Cochrane Database Syst Rev. 2016;12:CD010263.

112.   Yi J, Xiao J, Li H, Li Y, Li X, Zhao Z. Effectiveness of adjunctive interventions for accelerating orthodontic tooth movement: a systematic review of systematic reviews. J Oral Rehabil. 2017;44(8):636-654.

113.   Brosseau L, Welch V, Wells G, et al. Low level laser therapy for osteoarthritis and rheumatoid arthritis: a metaanalysis. J Rheumatol. 2000;27(8):1961-9.

114.   Jang H, Lee H. Meta-analysis of pain relief effects by laser irradiation on joint areas. Photomed Laser Surg. 2012;30(8):405-17.

115.   Bjordal JM, Johnson MI, Lopes-martins RA, Bogen B, Chow R, Ljunggren AE. Short-term efficacy of physical interventions in osteoarthritic knee pain. A systematic review and meta-analysis of randomised placebo-controlled trials. BMC Musculoskelet Disord. 2007;8:51.

116.   De souza merli LA, De medeiros VP, Toma L, et al. The low level laser therapy effect on the remodeling of bone extracellular matrix. Photochem Photobiol. 2012;88(5):1293-301.

117.   Saad A, El yamany M, Abbas O, Yehia M. Possible role of low level laser therapy on bone turnover in ovariectomized rats. Endocr Regul. 2010;44(4):155-63.

118.   Falaki F, Nejat AH, Dalirsani Z. The Effect of Low-level Laser Therapy on Trigeminal Neuralgia: A Review of Literature. J Dent Res Dent Clin Dent Prospects. 2014;8(1):1-5.

119.   Bjordal JM, Johnson MI, Iversen V, Aimbire F, Lopez-Martins RAB. Low-level laser therapy in acute pain: A systematic review of possible mechanisms of action and clinical effects in randomized placebo-controlled trials. Photomed Laser Surg. 2006; 24(2):158-168.

120.   Ren C, Mcgrath C, Jin L, Zhang C, Yang Y. The effectiveness of low-level laser therapy as an adjunct to non-surgical periodontal treatment: a meta-analysis. J Periodont Res. 2017;52(1):8-20.

121.   Chen YT, Wang HH, Wang TJ, Li YC, Chen TJ. Early application of low-level laser may

reduce the incidence of postherpetic neuralgia (PHN). J Am Acad Dermatol. 2016;75(3):572-577.

122.   Schubert V. Effects of phototherapy on pressure ulcer healing in elderly patients after a falling trauma. A prospective, randomized, controlled study. Photodermatol Photoimmunol Photomed. 2001;17(1):32-8.

123.   Dehlin O, Elmståhl S, Gottrup F. Monochromatic phototherapy: effective treatment for grade II chronic pressure ulcers in elderly patients. Aging Clin Exp Res. 2007;19(6):478-83.

124.   Costa MM, Silva SB, Quinto AL, et al. Phototherapy 660 nm for the prevention of radiodermatitis in breast cancer patients receiving radiation therapy: study protocol for a randomized controlled trial. Trials. 2014;15:330.

125.   Censabella S, Claes S, Robijns J, Bulens P, Mebis J. Photobiomodulation for the management of radiation dermatitis: the DERMIS trial, a pilot study of MLS(®) laser therapy in breast cancer patients. Support Care Cancer. 2016;24(9):3925-33.

126.   Strouthos I, Chatzikonstantinou G, Tselis N, et al. Photobiomodulation therapy for the management of radiation-induced dermatitis : A single-institution experience of adjuvant radiotherapy in breast cancer patients after breast conserving surgery. Strahlenther Onkol. 2017;193(6):491-498.

127.   Hirschl M, Katzenschlager R, Francesconi C, Kundi M. Low level laser therapy in primary Raynaud's phenomenon--results of a placebo

controlled, double blind intervention study. J Rheumatol. 2004;31(12):2408-12.

128. Derkacz A, Protasiewicz M, Poreba R, Szuba A, Andrzejak R. Usefulness of intravascular low-power laser illumination in preventing restenosis after percutaneous coronary intervention. Am J Cardiol. 2010;106(8):1113-7.

129. Brosseau L, Welch V, Wells G, et al. Low level laser therapy (classes I, II and III) in the treatment of rheumatoid arthritis. Cochrane Database Syst Rev. 2000;(2):CD002049.

130. Brosseau L, Robinson V, Wells G, et al. Low level laser therapy (Classes I, II and III) for treating rheumatoid arthritis. Cochrane Database Syst Rev. 2005;(4):CD002049.

131. Brosseau L, Welch V, Wells G, et al. Low level laser therapy for osteoarthritis and rheumatoid arthritis: a metaanalysis. J Rheumatol. 2000;27(8):1961-9.

132. Haslerud S, Magnussen LH, Joensen J, Lopes-martins RA, Bjordal JM. The efficacy of low-level laser therapy for shoulder tendinopathy: a systematic review and meta-analysis of randomized controlled trials. Physiother Res Int. 2015;20(2):108-25.

133. Lee SY, Park KH, Choi JW, et al. A prospective, randomized, placebo-controlled, double-blinded, and split-face clinical study on LED phototherapy for skin rejuvenation: clinical, profilometric, histologic, ultrastructural, and biochemical evaluations and comparison of three

different treatment settings. J Photochem Photobiol B, Biol. 2007;88(1):51-67.

134. Calderhead RG, Kim WS, Ohshiro T, Trelles MA, Vasily DB. Adjunctive 830 nm light-emitting diode therapy can improve the results following aesthetic procedures. Laser Ther. 2015;24(4):277-89.

135. De oliveira RA, Fernandes GA, Lima AC, Tajra filho AD, De barros araújo R, Nicolau RA. The effects of LED emissions on sternotomy incision repair after myocardial revascularization: a randomized double-blind study with follow-up. Lasers Med Sci. 2014;29(3):1195-202.

136. Fernandes GA, Lima AC, Gonzaga IC, De barros araújo R, De oliveira RA, Nicolau RA. Low-intensity laser (660 nm) on sternotomy healing in patients who underwent coronary artery bypass graft: a randomized, double-blind study. Lasers Med Sci. 2016;31(9):1907-1913.

137. Lima AC, Fernandes GA, De barros araújo R, Gonzaga IC, De oliveira RA, Nicolau RA. Photobiomodulation (Laser and LED) on Sternotomy Healing in Hyperglycemic and Normoglycemic Patients Who Underwent Coronary Bypass Surgery with Internal Mammary Artery Grafts: A Randomized, Double-Blind Study with Follow-Up. Photomed Laser Surg. 2017;35(1):24-31.

138. Yip S, Zivin J. Laser therapy in acute stroke treatment. Int J Stroke. 2008;3(2):88-91.

139.   Lapchak PA. Taking a light approach to treating acute ischemic stroke patients: transcranial near-infrared laser therapy translational science. Ann Med. 2010;42(8):576-86.

140.   Lapchak PA, Boitano PD. Transcranial Near-Infrared Laser Therapy for Stroke: How to Recover from Futility in the NEST-3 Clinical Trial. Acta Neurochir Suppl. 2016;121:7-12.

141.   Barolet D, Boucher A. LED photoprevention: reduced MED response following multiple LED exposures. Lasers Surg Med. 2008;40(2):106-12.

142.   Chen J, Huang Z, Ge M, Gao M. Efficacy of low-level laser therapy in the treatment of TMDs: a meta-analysis of 14 randomised controlled trials. J Oral Rehabil. 2015;42(4):291-9.

143.   Tumilty S, Munn J, Mcdonough S, Hurley DA, Basford JR, Baxter GD. Low level laser treatment of tendinopathy: a systematic review with meta-analysis. Photomed Laser Surg. 2010;28(1):3-16.

144.   Ahn JC, Kim YH, Rhee CK. The effects of low level laser therapy (LLLT) on the testis in elevating serum testosterone level in rats. 24(1): 28-32.

145.   Souza LW, Souza SV, Botelho AC. Endonyx toenail onychomycosis caused by Trichophyton rubrum: treatment with photodynamic therapy based on methylene blue dye. An Bras Dermatol. 2013;88(6):1019-21.

146.   Souza LW, Souza SV, Botelho AC. Distal and lateral toenail onychomycosis caused by Trichophyton rubrum: treatment with photodynamic therapy based on methylene blue dye. An Bras Dermatol. 2014;89(1):184-6.

147.   Robres P, Aspiroz C, Rezusta A, Gilaberte Y. Usefulness of Photodynamic Therapy in the Management of Onychomycosis. Actas Dermosifiliogr. 2015;106(10):795-805.

148.   Naeser MA, Zafonte R, Krengel MH, et al. Significant improvements in cognitive performance post-transcranial, red/near-infrared light-emitting diode treatments in chronic, mild traumatic brain injury: open-protocol study. J Neurotrauma. 2014;31(11):1008-17.

149.   Naeser MA, Martin PI, Ho MD, et al. Transcranial, Red/Near-Infrared Light-Emitting Diode Therapy to Improve Cognition in Chronic Traumatic Brain Injury. Photomed Laser Surg. 2016;34(12):610-626.

150.   Gupta AK, Filonenko N, Salansky N, Sauder DN. The use of low energy photon therapy (LEPT) in venous leg ulcers: a double-blind, placebo-controlled study. Dermatol Surg. 1998;24(12):1383-6.

151.   Wu CS, Hu SC, Lan CC, Chen GS, Chuo WH, Yu HS. Low-energy helium-neon laser therapy induces repigmentation and improves the abnormalities of cutaneous microcirculation in segmental-type vitiligo lesions. Kaohsiung J Med Sci. 2008;24(4):180-9.

152.   Lan CC, Wu CS, Chiou MH, Chiang TY, Yu HS. Low-energy helium-neon laser induces melanocyte proliferation via interaction with type IV collagen: visible light as a therapeutic option for vitiligo. Br J Dermatol. 2009;161(2):273-80.

153.   Hopkins JT, Mcloda TA, Seegmiller JG, David baxter G. Low-Level Laser Therapy Facilitates Superficial Wound Healing in Humans: A Triple-Blind, Sham-Controlled Study. J Athl Train. 2004;39(3):223-229.

154.   Krynicka I, Rutowski R, Staniszewska-kuś J, Fugiel J, Zaleski A. The role of laser biostimulation in early post-surgery rehabilitation and its effect on wound healing. Ortop Traumatol Rehabil. 2010;12(1):67-79.

155.   Lins RD, Dantas EM, Lucena KC, Catão MH, Granville-garcia AF, Carvalho neto LG. Biostimulation effects of low-power laser in the repair process. An Bras Dermatol. 2010;85(6):849-55.

TOP 10 PROVEN BENEFITS OF RED LIGHT

1. "Overweight & Obesity." Centers for Disease Control and Prevention. (2017). Available: https://www.cdc.gov/obesity/data/adult.html [February 10, 2018].

2. Sene-fiorese M, Duarte FO, De aquino junior AE, et al. The potential of phototherapy to reduce body fat, insulin resistance and "metabolic inflexibility" related to obesity in women

undergoing weight loss treatment. Lasers Surg Med. 2015;47(8):634-42.

3. Duarte FO, Sene-fiorese M, De aquino junior AE, et al. Can low-level laser therapy (LLLT) associated with an aerobic plus resistance training change the cardiometabolic risk in obese women? A placebo-controlled clinical trial. J Photochem Photobiol B, Biol. 2015;153:103-10.

4. Nestor MS, Newburger J, Zarraga MB. Body contouring using 635-nm low level laser therapy. Semin Cutan Med Surg. 2013;32(1):35-40.

5. Jackson RF, Dedo DD, Roche GC, Turok DI, Maloney RJ. Low-level laser therapy as a non-invasive approach for body contouring: a randomized, controlled study. Lasers Surg Med. 2009;41(10):799-809.

6. Mcrae E, Boris J. Independent evaluation of low-level laser therapy at 635 nm for non-invasive body contouring of the waist, hips, and thighs. Lasers Surg Med. 2013;45(1):1-7.

7. NASA press release (2000). NASA Space Technology Shines Light on Healing. [Online]. Available: http://www.laserthera.com/press_release_3.htm [August 1st, 2017].

8. Hopkins JT, Mcloda TA, Seegmiller JG, David baxter G. Low-Level Laser Therapy Facilitates Superficial Wound Healing in Humans: A Triple-Blind, Sham-Controlled Study. J Athl Train. 2004;39(3):223-229.

9. Chaves ME de A, de Araújo AR, Piancastelli ACC, Pinotti M. Effects of low-power light therapy on wound healing: LASER x LED . *Anais Brasileiros de Dermatologia*. 2014;89(4):616-623.

10. Barbosa D, De souza RA, Xavier M, Da silva FF, Arisawa EA, Villaverde AG. Effects of low-level laser therapy (LLLT) on bone repair in rats: optical densitometry analysis. Lasers Med Sci. 2013;28(2):651-6.

11. Pinheiro AL, Limeira júnior Fde A, Gerbi ME, Ramalho LM, Marzola C, Ponzi EA. Effect of low level laser therapy on the repair of bone defects grafted with inorganic bovine bone. Braz Dent J. 2003;14(3):177-81.

12. Pinheiro AL, Gerbi ME. Photoengineering of bone repair processes. Photomed Laser Surg. 2006;24(2):169-78.

13. Blaya DS, Guimarães MB, Pozza DH, Weber JB, De oliveira MG. Histologic study of the effect of laser therapy on bone repair. J Contemp Dent Pract. 2008;9(6):41-8.

14. The Healthline Editorial Team, Gotter A and Rogers G, MD. Low Testosterone in Men. Healthline. Jul 2016.

15. Andre B. Araujo, Gretchen R. Esche, Varant Kupelian, Amy B. O'Donnell, Thomas G. Travison, Rachel E. Williams, Richard V. Clark, John B. McKinlay; Prevalence of Symptomatic Androgen Deficiency in Men, *The Journal of Clinical Endocrinology & Metabolism*, Volume 92, Issue 11, 1 November 2007, Pages 4241–4247.

16. Ahn JC, Kim YH, Rhee CK. The effects of low level laser therapy (LLLT) on the testis in elevating serum testosterone level in rats. Biomed Res. 2013;24(1):28-32.

17. Barrett DW, Gonzalez-lima F. Transcranial infrared laser stimulation produces beneficial cognitive and emotional effects in humans. Neuroscience. 2013;230:13-23.

18. Hwang J, Castelli DM, Gonzalez-lima F. Cognitive enhancement by transcranial laser stimulation and acute aerobic exercise. Lasers Med Sci. 2016;31(6):1151-60.

19. Reddy MS. Depression: the disorder and the burden. Indian J Psychol Med. 2010;32(1):1-2.

20. Weissman JD, Russel D, Jay M, Beasley JM, Malaspina D, Pegus C. Disparities in Health Care Utilization and Functional Limitations Among Adults with Serious Psychological Distress, 2006-2014. *Psych. Serv.* 2016;68(7):653-659.

21. Ibrahim AK, Kelly SJ, Adams CE, Glazebrook C. A systematic review of studies of depression prevalence in university students. J Psychiatr Res. 2013;47(3):391-400.

22. Facts & Statistics. Anxiety and Depression Association of America. [Online]. Available: https://adaa.org/about-adaa/press-room/facts-statistics [August 1, 2017].

23. Schiffer F, Johnston AL, Ravichandran C, et al. Psychological benefits 2 and 4 weeks after a single treatment with near infrared light to the forehead:

a pilot study of 10 patients with major depression and anxiety. Behav Brain Funct. 2009;5:46.

24. Bickers DR, Lim HW, Margolis D, Weinstock MA, Goodman C, Faulkner E et al. The burden of skin diseases: 2004 a joint project of the American Academy of Dermatology Association and the Society for Investigative Dermatology.Journal of the American Academy of Dermatology 2006;55:490-500.

25. Strauss JS, Krowchuk DP, Leyden JJ, Lucky AW, Shalita AR, Siegfried EC et al. Guidelines of care for acne vulgaris management. Journal of the American Academy of Dermatology 2007;56:651-63.

26. Smithard A, Glazebrook C, Williams HC. Acne prevalence, knowledge about acne and psychological morbidity in mid-adolescence: a community-based study. Br J Dermatol. 2001;145(2):274-9.

27. Aziz-jalali MH, Tabaie SM, Djavid GE. Comparison of Red and Infrared Low-level Laser Therapy in the Treatment of Acne Vulgaris. Indian J Dermatol. 2012;57(2):128-30.

28. Richard L. Nahin. Estimates of Pain Prevalence and Severity in Adults: United States, 2012. *The Journal of Pain*, 2015; 16 (8): 769.

29. FDA Drug Safety Communication: FDA strengthens warning that non-aspirin nonsteroidal anti-inflammatory drugs (NSAIDs) can cause heart attacks or strokes. 2015. Available:

https://www.fda.gov/Drugs/DrugSafety/ucm451
800.htm [August 10, 2017].

30. Bjordal JM, Johnson MI, Iversen V, Aimbire F, Lopes-martins RA. Low-level laser therapy in acute pain: a systematic review of possible mechanisms of action and clinical effects in randomized placebo-controlled trials. Photomed Laser Surg. 2006;24(2):158-68.

31. Chow RT, Johnson MI, Lopes-martins RA, Bjordal JM. Efficacy of low-level laser therapy in the management of neck pain: a systematic review and meta-analysis of randomised placebo or active-treatment controlled trials. Lancet. 2009;374(9705):1897-908.

32. Falaki F, Nejat AH, Dalirsani Z. The Effect of Low-level Laser Therapy on Trigeminal Neuralgia: A Review of Literature. J Dent Res Dent Clin Dent Prospects. 2014;8(1):1-5.

33. Avci P, Gupta GK, Clark J, Wikonkal N, Hamblin MR. Low-level laser (light) therapy (LLLT) for treatment of hair loss. Lasers Surg Med. 2014;46(2):144-51.

34. Statistic Brain. Hair Loss Statistics. 2016. Available: http://www.statisticbrain.com/hair-loss-statistics [August 20th, 2017].

35. Jain, R. et al. Potential targets in the discovery of new hair growth promoters for androgenic alopecia. July 2014, Vol. 18, No. 7 , Pages 787-806.

36. Danny Roddy. 2014. Hair Like a Fox: A bioenergetics view of pattern h air loss frequently asked questions. Available:

http://www.dannyroddy.com/weblog/hairlikeafo
xfaq [August 25, 2017].

37. Arthritis-Related Statistics. Centers for disease
Control and Prevention. Available:
https://www.cdc.gov/arthritis/data_statistics/arth
ritis-related-stats.htm [August 20, 2017].

38. Hamblin MR. Can osteoarthritis be treated with
light? Arthritis Res. & Ther. 2013;15:120.

LIGHT THERAPY FOR CANCER

1. Seyfried TN, Shelton LM. Cancer as a metabolic
disease. Nutr Metab (Lond). 2010;7:7.

2. The cancer genome. Nature. 2009;458(7239):719.

3. Mandinova A, Lee SW. The p53 pathway as a
target in cancer therapeutics: obstacles and
promise. Sci Transl Med. 2011;3(64):64rv1.

4. Gravendeel LA, Kouwenhoven MC, Gevaert O, et
al. Intrinsic gene expression profiles of gliomas are
a better predictor of survival than histology.
Cancer Res. 2009;69(23):9065-72.

5. Dang L, White DW, Gross S, et al. Cancer-
associated IDH1 mutations produce 2-
hydroxyglutarate. Nature. 2009;462(7274):739-44.

6. Warburg O. Uber den Stoffwechsel der
Hefe.pp252-254.

How Does Red Light Heal?

1. Bianconi E, Piovesan A, Facchin F, et al. An estimation of the number of cells in the human body. Ann Hum Biol. 2013;40(6):463-71.

2. Otto Warburg. Otto-Warburg-Medal. Available: http://otto-warburg-medal.org/index.php/otto-warburg-30.html [February 10, 2018].

3. Yonetani T, Ray GS. Studies on Cytochrome Oxidase. 1965; 240(8): 3392-3398.

4. Li, Y., Park, JS., Deng, JH. et al. Cytochrome c oxidase subunit IV is essential for assembly and respiratory function of the enzyme complex. J Bioenerg Biomembr (2006) 38: 283.

5. Herrmann, P.C. & Herrmann, E.C. Oxygen Metabolism and a potential role for cytochrome c oxidase in the Warburg effect. J Bioenerg Biomembr (2007) 39: 247.

6. Dong DW, Srinivasan S, Guha M, Avadhani NG. Defects in cytochrome c oxidase expression induce a metabolic shift to glycolysis and carcinogenesis. Genom Data. 2015;6:99-107.

7. Brian B. Hasinoff, John P. Davey & Peter J. O'brien (2009) The Adriamycin (doxorubicin)-induced inactivation of cytochrome c oxidase depends on the presence of iron or copper, Xenobiotica, 19:2, 231-241.

8. Stannard JN, Horecker BL. The in vitro inhibition of cytochrome oxidase by azide and cyanide. J biol chem. 1947; 172: 599-608.

9. Wilson MT, Antonini G, Malatesta F, Sarti P, Brunori M. Probing the oxygen binding site of cytochrome c oxidase by cyanide. J Biol Chem. 1994;269(39):24114-9.

10. Jensen P, Wilson MT, Aasa R, Malmström BG. Cyanide inhibition of cytochrome c oxidase. A rapid-freeze e.p.r. investigation. Biochem J. 1984;224(3):829-37.

11. Miró O, Casademont J, Barrientos A, Urbano-márquez A, Cardellach F. Mitochondrial cytochrome c oxidase inhibition during acute carbon monoxide poisoning. Pharmacol Toxicol. 1998;82(4):199-202.

12. Carbon Monoxide Specifically Inhibits Cytochrome C Oxidase of Human Mitochondrial Respiratory Chain. Basic & Clinical Pharmacology. Toxicology. 2003; 93(3):142.

13. Amores E, Forde-baker J, Ginsburg BY, Nelson LS. Cytochrome-C oxidase inhibition in 26 aluminum phosphide poisoned patients. Clin Toxicol (Phila). 2007;45(5):461.

14. Kotwicka M, Skibinska I, Jendraszak M, Jedrezejczak P. 17b-estradiol modifies human spermatozoa mitochondrial function in vitro. Reprod Biol Endocrinol. 2016; 14:50.

15. Harvey AT, Preskorn SH. Cytochrome P450 enzymes: interpretation of their interactions with selective serotonin reuptake inhibitors. Part II. J Clin Psychopharmacol. 1996;16(5):345-55.

16. Levy RJ, Vijayasarathy C, Raj NR, Avadhani NG, Deutschman CS. Competitive and noncompetitive

inhibition of myocardial cytochrome C oxidase in sepsis. Shock. 2004;21(2):110-4.

17. Nagai N, Ito Y. Dysfunction in cytochrome c oxidase caused by excessive nitric oxide in human lens epithelial cells stimulated with interferon-γ and lipopolysaccharide. Curr Eye Res. 2012;37(10):889-97.

18. Mohapatra NK, Roberts JF. In vitro effect of aflatoxin B1 on rat liver macrophages (Kuffer cells). Toxicol Lett. 1985;29(2-3):177-81.

19. Oriowo OM. Fluorometric Quantitation of Cytochrome C Oxidase Activity in Cultured Crystalline Lenses. Inv Ophth & Vis Sci. 2003; 44(13):305.

20. Warburg O. On the Origin of Cancer Cells. Science. 1956; 123: 309-14.

21. Zhong J, Rajaram N, Brizel DM, et al. Radiation induces aerobic glycolysis through reactive oxygen species. Radiother Oncol. 2013;106(3):390-6.

22. Kunkel HO, Williams JN. The effects of fat deficiency upon enzyme activity in the rat. J Biol Chem. 1951;189(2):755-61.

23. Brown GC, Cooper CE. Nanomolar concentrations of nitric oxide reversibly inhibit synaptosomal respiration by competing with oxygen at cytochrome oxidase. FEBS letters. 1994; 356(2-3): 295-298.

24. Bolanos JP, Peuchen S, Heales SJR, Land JM, Clark JB. Nitric Oxide- Mediated Inhibition of the Mitochondrial Respiratory Chain in Cultured

Astrocytes. Journal of Neurochemistry. 1994; 63(3):910.

25. Cleeter MW, Cooper JM, Darley-usmar VM, Moncada S, Schapira AH. Reversible inhibition of cytochrome c oxidase, the terminal enzyme of the mitochondrial respiratory chain, by nitric oxide. Implications for neurodegenerative diseases. FEBS Lett. 1994;345(1):50-4.

26. Brown GC, Borutaite V. Nitric oxide, cytochrome c and mitochondria. Biochem Soc Symp. 1999;66:17-25.

27. Hamblin MR. The role of nitric oxide in low level light therapy. SPIE. 2008; 6846.

28. Hamblin MR, Demidova TN. Mechanisms of low level light therapy. Int Soc Opt Eng. 2006; 6140:1-12.

29. Karu T, Tiphlova O, Esenaliev R, Letokhov V. Two different mechanisms of low-intensity laser photobiological effects on Escherichia coli. J Photochem Photobiol B, Biol. 1994;24(3):155-61.

30. Morimoto Y, Arai T, Kikuchi M, Nakajima S, Nakamura H. Effect of low-intensity argon laser irradiation on mitochondrial respiration. Lasers Surg Med. 1994;15(2):191-9.

31. Passarella S, Ostuni A, Atlante A, Quagliariello E. Increase in the ADP/ATP exchange in rat liver mitochondria irradiated in vitro by helium-neon laser. Biochem Biophys Res Commun. 1988;156(2):978-86.

32. Greco M, Guida G, Perlino E, Marra E, Quagliariello E. Increase in RNA and protein synthesis by mitochondria irradiated with helium-neon laser. Biochem Biophys Res Commun. 1989;163(3):1428-34.

33. Karu T, Pyatibrat L, Kalendo G. Irradiation with HeNe laser increases ATP level in cells cultivated in vitro. J Photochem Photobiol. 1995; 27(3):219-223.

34. Pastore D, Martino CD, Bosco G, Passarella S. Stimulation of ATP synthesis via oxidative phosphorylation in wheat mitochondria irradiated with helium-neon laser. Life. 1996; 39(1):149-157.

35. Pastore D, Greco M, Passarella S. Specific helium-neon laser sensitivity of the purified cytochrome c oxidase. Int J Radiat Biol. 2000;76(6):863-70.

36. Karu T. Primary and secondary mechanisms of action of visible to near-IR radiation on cells. J Photochem Photobiol B, Biol. 1999;49(1):1-17.

37. Eells JT, Henry MM, Summerfelt P, et al. Therapeutic photobiomodulation for methanol-induced retinal toxicity. Proc Natl Acad Sci USA. 2003;100(6):3439-44.

38. Karu TI, Pyatibrat LV, Ryabykh TP. Melatonin modulates the action of near infrared radiation on cell adhesion. Journal of Pineal Research. 2003;34(3):167.

39. Karu TI, Pyatibrat LV, Kalendo GS. Photobiological modulation of cell attachment via cytochrome c oxidase. Photochem Photobiol Sci. 2004;3(2):211-6.

40. Eells JT, Wong-riley MT, Verhoeve J, et al. Mitochondrial signal transduction in accelerated wound and retinal healing by near-infrared light therapy. Mitochondrion. 2004;4(5-6):559-67.

41. Karu TI, Pyatibrat LV, Afanasyeva NI. Cellular effects of low power laser therapy can be mediated by nitric oxide. Lasers Surg Med. 2005;36(4):307-14.

42. Karu TI, Pyatibrat LV, Kolyakov SF, Afanasyeva NI. Absorption measurements of a cell monolayer relevant to phototherapy: reduction of cytochrome c oxidase under near IR radiation. J Photochem Photobiol B, Biol. 2005;81(2):98-106.

43. Karu TI, Kolyakov SF. Exact action spectra for cellular responses relevant to phototherapy. Photomed Laser Surg. 2005;23(4):355-61.

44. Wong-riley MT, Liang HL, Eells JT, et al. Photobiomodulation directly benefits primary neurons functionally inactivated by toxins: role of cytochrome c oxidase. J Biol Chem. 2005;280(6):4761-71.

45. Yeager RL, Franzosa JA, Millsap DS, et al. Survivorship and mortality implications of developmental 670-nm phototherapy: dioxin co-exposure. Photomed Laser Surg. 2006;24(1):29-32.

46. Liang HL, Whelan HT, Eells JT, et al. Photobiomodulation partially rescues visual cortical neurons from cyanide-induced apoptosis. Neuroscience. 2006;139(2):639-49.

47. Chung H, Dai T, Sharma SK, Huang YY, Carroll JD, Hamblin MR. The nuts and bolts of low-level

laser (light) therapy. Ann Biomed Eng. 2012;40(2):516-33.

48. Prindeze NJ, Moffatt LT, Shupp JW. Mechanisms of action for light therapy: a review of molecular interactions. Exp Biol Med (Maywood). 2012;237(11):1241-8.

49. Karu T. Primary and secondary mechanisms of action of visible to near-IR radiation on cells. J Photochem Photobiol B, Biol. 1999;49(1):1-17.

50. De freitas LF, Hamblin MR. Proposed Mechanisms of Photobiomodulation or Low-Level Light Therapy. IEEE J Sel Top Quantum Electron. 2016;22(3).

51. Oxidative Phosphorylation: Definition, Steps & Products. Study.com. Available: https://study.com/academy/lesson/oxidative-phosphorylation-definition-steps-products.html [February 10, 2018].

52. Kilmartin JV. The Bohr effect of human hemoglobin. Trends in Bio. Sci. 1977;2(11):247-249.

53. Tyuma I. The Bohr effect and the Haldane effect in human hemoglobin. Jpn J Physiol. 1984;34(2):205-16.

54. Poyart CF, Bursaux E. [Current conception of the Bohr effect]. Poumon Coeur. 1975;31(4):173-7.

55. Frangez I, Cankar K, Ban frangez H, Smrke DM. The effect of LED on blood microcirculation during chronic wound healing in diabetic and non-diabetic patients-a prospective, double-blind

randomized study. Lasers Med Sci. 2017;32(4):887-894.

56. Podogrodzki J, Lebiedowski M, Szalecki M, Kępa I, Syczewska M, Jóźwiak S. [Impact of low level laser therapy on skin blood flow]. Dev Period Med. 2016;20(1):40-6.

57. Fouda AA, Refai H, Mohammed NH. Low level laser therapy versus pulsed electromagnetic field for inactivation of myofascial trigger points. A J Res Comm. 2013; 1(3):68-78.

58. Andre ES, Dalmarco EM, Gomes LEA. The brain-derived neurotrophic factor nerve growth factor, neurotrophin-3, and induced nitric oxide synthase expression after low-level laser therapy in an axonotmesis experimental model. Photomed laser surg. 2012; 30(11):1-6.

59. Yeager RL, Lim J, Millsap DS, et al. 670 nanometer light treatment attenuates dioxin toxicity in the developing chick embryo. J Biochem Mol Toxicol. 2006;20(6):271-8.

60. Lim J, Sanders RA, Yeager RL, et al. Attenuation of TCDD-induced oxidative stress by 670 nm photobiomodulation in developmental chicken kidney. J Biochem Mol Toxicol. 2008;22(4):230-9.

61. Silva macedo R, Peres leal M, Braga TT, et al. Photobiomodulation Therapy Decreases Oxidative Stress in the Lung Tissue after Formaldehyde Exposure: Role of Oxidant/Antioxidant Enzymes. Mediators Inflamm. 2016;2016:9303126.

62. Dos santos SA, Serra AJ, Stancker TG, et al. Effects of Photobiomodulation Therapy on

Oxidative Stress in Muscle Injury Animal Models: A Systematic Review. Oxid Med Cell Longev. 2017;2017:5273403.

63. Hamblin MR. Mechanisms and applications of the anti-inflammatory effects of photobiomodulation. AIMS Biophys. 2017;4(3):337-361.

64. Denadai AS, Aydos RD, Silva IS, et al. Acute effects of low-level laser therapy (660 nm) on oxidative stress levels in diabetic rats with skin wounds. J Exp Ther Oncol. 2017;11(2):85-89.

Is Red Light Therapy Safe?

1. Dr Michael Hamblin: Harvard Professor and Infrared Therapy Expert: Michael Hamblin, 2015. SelfHacked. YouTube. Available: https://www.youtube.com/watch?v=wAW8Fvg-TJQ. [January 31, 2018].

2. Basford JR, Cheville AL. An assessment of the role of low-level laser therapy in the treatment of lymphedema. Dermanova. Available: http://dermanova.spdev.co.nz/images/custom/laser_therapy_article_4.pdf [February 10, 2018].

Two Proven Ways to Accelerate Healing

1. Mandal MD, Mandal S. Honey: its medicinal property and antibacterial activity. Asian Pac J Trop Biomed. 2011;1(2):154-60.

2. Gupta SS, Singh O, Bhagel PS, Moses S, Shukla S, Mathur RK. Honey dressing versus silver sulfadiazene dressing for wound healing in burn

patients: a retrospective study. J Cutan Aesthet Surg. 2011;4(3):183-7.

3. Yadav A, Verma S, Keshri GK, Gupta A. Combination of medicinal honey and 904□nm superpulsed laser-mediated photobiomodulation promotes healing and impedes inflammation, pain in full-thickness burn. J Photochem Photobiol B, Biol. 2018;186:152-159.

4. Shilling M, Matt L, Rubin E, et al. Antimicrobial effects of virgin coconut oil and its medium-chain fatty acids on Clostridium difficile. J Med Food. 2013;16(12):1079-85.

5. Verallo-rowell VM, Dillague KM, Syah-tjundawan BS. Novel antibacterial and emollient effects of coconut and virgin olive oils in adult atopic dermatitis. Dermatitis. 2008;19(6):308-15.

6. Shino B, Peedikayil FC, Jaiprakash SR, Ahmed bijapur G, Kottayi S, Jose D. Comparison of Antimicrobial Activity of Chlorhexidine, Coconut Oil, Probiotics, and Ketoconazole on Candida albicans Isolated in Children with Early Childhood Caries: An In Vitro Study. Scientifica (Cairo). 2016;2016:7061587.

7. Ogbolu DO, Oni AA, Daini OA, Oloko AP. In vitro antimicrobial properties of coconut oil on Candida species in Ibadan, Nigeria. J Med Food. 2007;10(2):384-7.

8. Coconut oil in health and disease: Its and monolaurin's potential as cure for aids. Unknown journal. Date unknown. Available: https://www.researchgate.net/publication/237233

256_COCONUT_OIL_IN_HEALTH_AND_DI
SEASE_ITS_AND_MONOLAURIN%27S_POT
ENTIAL_AS_CURE_FOR_HIVAIDS_By.
[February 15, 2017].

9. Interviews and anecdotal reports. Posit Health News. 1998;(No 16):13-5.

10. Nevin KG, Rajamohan T. Effect of topical application of virgin coconut oil on skin components and antioxidant status during dermal wound healing in young rats. Skin Pharmacol Physiol. 2010;23(6):290-7.

11. Steinbrenner I, Houdek P, Pollok S, Brandner JM, Daniels R. Influence of the Oil Phase and Topical Formulation on the Wound Healing Ability of a Birch Bark Dry Extract. PLoS ONE. 2016;11(5).

YOUR QUESTIONS ANSWERED

1. Yadav A, Gupta A, Keshri GK, Verma S, Sharma SK, Singh SB. Photobiomodulatory effects of superpulsed 904nm laser therapy on bioenergetics status in burn wound healing. J Photochem Photobiol B, Biol. 2016;162:77-85.

2. Gupta A, Keshri GK, Yadav A, et al. Superpulsed (Ga-As, 904 nm) low-level laser therapy (LLLT) attenuates inflammatory response and enhances healing of burn wounds. J Biophotonics. 2015;8(6):489-501.

3. Al-watban FA, Zhang XY. The comparison of effects between pulsed and CW lasers on wound healing. J Clin Laser Med Surg. 2004;22(1):15-8.

4. Keshri GK, Gupta A, Yadav A, Sharma SK, Singh SB. Photobiomodulation with Pulsed and Continuous Wave Near-Infrared Laser (810 nm, Al-Ga-As) Augments Dermal Wound Healing in Immunosuppressed Rats. PLoS ONE. 2016;11(11):e0166705.

5. Joensen J, Ovsthus K, Reed RK, et al. Skin penetration time-profiles for continuous 810 nm and Superpulsed 904 nm lasers in a rat model. Photomed Laser Surg. 2012;30(12):688-94.

6. Ando T, Xuan W, Xu T, et al. Comparison of therapeutic effects between pulsed and continuous wave 810-nm wavelength laser irradiation for traumatic brain injury in mice. PLoS ONE. 2011;6(10):e26212.

7. Ilic S, Leichliter S, Streeter J, Oron A, Detaboada L, Oron U. Effects of power densities, continuous and pulse frequencies, and number of sessions of low-level laser therapy on intact rat brain. Photomed Laser Surg. 2006;24(4):458-66.

8. Keshri GK, Gupta A, Yadav A, Sharma SK, Singh SB. Photobiomodulation with Pulsed and Continuous Wave Near-Infrared Laser (810 nm, Al-Ga-As) Augments Dermal Wound Healing in Immunosuppressed Rats. PLoS ONE. 2016;11(11):e0166705.

INDEX

PLEASE REVIEW THIS!

I hope you enjoyed this book and that it has given you hope for a *brighter* future (pun intended) in which people can heal exceptionally well without using medicines that cause harm.

If this book helped or entertained you in any way, all I ask in return is that you take a moment to write an honest, sincere review of this book on Amazon. It will only take a few minutes, and it will help me out more than you can imagine.

To leave a review, search "Red light Mark Sloan" on Amazon to find the book page or visit the following link, then scroll down and write a couple of quick sentences:

AMAZON.COM/DP/0994741863

ABOUT THE AUTHOR

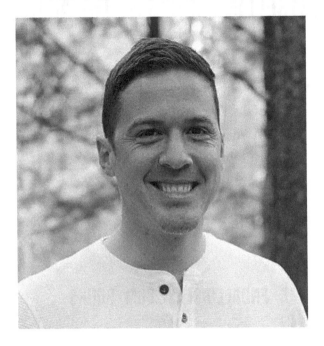

MARK SLOAN has written over 300 articles and is the author of *The Cancer Industry, Cancer: The Metabolic Disease Unravelled* and the 6x international #1 bestseller *Red Light Therapy: Miracle Medicine*. Mark lives in Ontario, Canada and his goal is to build an off grid home, raise a big, beautiful family and live a self-sufficient, resilient and responsible life as God had intended. Mark is passionate about learning and his ultimate goal in life is to reduce the suffering in this world and to make a better place for every human being alive and for future generations.

MORE INTERNATIONAL #1
BESTSELLING BOOKS BY THE AUTHOR

- The Cancer Industry
- Cancer: The Metabolic Disease Unravelled
- Red Light Therapy: Miracle Medicine
- The Ultimate Guide to Methylene Blue
- Bath Bombs & Balneotherapy
- And more!

Checkout all of Mark Sloan's books by visiting the following link:

ENDALLDISEASE.COM/BOOKS

A FREE GIFT FOR YOU

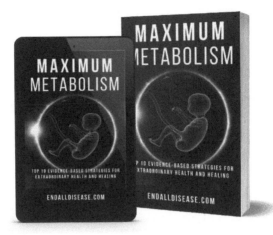

To say thanks for reading my book, I wanted to give you my groundbreaking ebook *Maximum Metabolism*, which includes the 10 most powerful evidence-based strategies for recovering from disease, improving overall health and extending lifespan, amassed from over 15 years of dedicated health research.

WWW.ENDALLDISEASE.COM/SPECIALOFFER

FREE GIFT #2: RED LIGHT THERAPY VIDEO COURSE

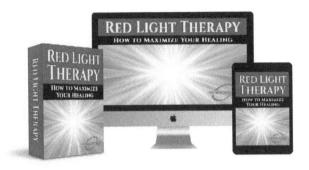

Want to know what Red Light Therapy can do for your health and how to get remarkable results from home?

Watch the world's first Red Light Therapy Video Course by #1 Bestselling Author of Red Light Therapy: Miracle Medicine, for FREE at the link below:

WWW.ENDALLDISEASE.COM/SPECIALOFFER

PREMIUM QUALITY RED LIGHT THERAPY DEVICES... AT A DISCOUNT!

Unsure which red light to buy? Learn which red light therapy devices I use and recommend and get an exclusive discount code for your order.

Unlock exclusive Endalldisease Insider deals on red light therapy, methylene blue, balneotherapy, hormone therapy, CO2 therapy, and more, for FREE at the link below:

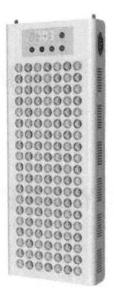

ENDALLDISEASE.COM/REDLIGHTUNLOCK